Keto Diet: The Risks and Benefits You Should Know First!

&

A Beginner's Guide to a Ketogenic Diet

Bonus!

Wouldn't it be to know when Amazon's top kindle books go on Free Promotion? Well now is your chance!

I would like to give you full access to an exclusive service that will email you notifications when Amazon' top Kindle books go on Free Promotion. If you are someone who is interested in saving a ton of money, then simply go to the link below for Free access.

https://bit.ly/2xFpfOX

As a "Thank you" for downloading this book, I would like to give you "30 Day Low Carb Diet Ketosis Plan" ebook to start your keto journey.

Introduction

What is a Keto Diet?

Key factors which make keto different

Taking care of our body and ourselves has always been a concern; however, the ways to maintain a healthy lifestyle are so highlighted in the modern world today. Many sources have thoroughly discussed the importance of eating a nutritious meal and exercising has always been one of the most crucial aspects. We may come across numerous diet plans and exercises to stay healthy and happy. One of the beneficial ways to do so is a keto diet. The ketones are produced in the liver by the body to use as energy in a low-carb diet. A keto diet is also referred to as a low-carb, high-fat (LCHF) diet.

Your body produces glucose and insulin when you eat a food rich in carbs. Glucose is chosen over any other source of energy, as it is the most natural molecule to convert in the form of heat. When our food intake is low, our body tends to help us in a natural process called ketosis. In this state, our body produces ketones from the breakdown of fats in the liver. Once you start undertaking a keto diet, your body becomes adaptive to it. There are many non-highlighted benefits of a keto diet, which helps you maintain your overall fitness.

Chapter 1: Ketosis

The process of ketosis in detail

By now, you must have already known that a ketogenic diet is a low-carb, high fat and moderate protein diet in which your body uses glucose as the primary source of energy. You can find this information based on an exciting premise which says that our collection was designed to run in a more efficient way as a fat burner than a sugar burner. The natural process of ketosis is when our food intake is low. When one lowers his/her carb intake, blood sugar levels, along with glucose levels, also drop resulting in reducing the insulin levels. Due to this, fat cells release the water they are storing, and then these cells can enter the bloodstream and head to the liver ultimately. That is the end goal of the ketogenic diet.

It is a myth that you enter into ketosis by starving your body. Instead, you come into ketosis by dying your body of carbohydrates. Since the fuel supply of your body switches to fats and insulin levels are deficient, burning fat becomes very easy. It starts utilizing your stored fat as it becomes accessible. That helps you in getting a steady supply of energy. To remain in ketosis, net carbs lower than 100g are advisable. Your diet will be as effective as you lower your carb intake. One must try to entirely avoid foods having starch and sugar while being on a ketogenic diet. One may begin to notice weight loss and physical and mental health improvement when his/her body is producing optimal ketone levels.

Chapter 2: Benefits of a Keto Diet

Fundamental ways in which a keto diet can help you

The word keto in 'ketogenic diet' is present because it makes our body produce small fuel particles termed as ketones. The body uses them when the blood sugar or glucose is in very short supply. One can accurately term them as the alternative fuel. As already discussed, the body produces ketones when one has a regulated intake of carbs that are broken down into blood sugar quickly and moderate proteins. Ketones, thus, develop in the liver from fat. After being produced, they are used as fuel throughout the body, including the brain. The brain is an organ, which requires energy the whole day and every day. It is a very hungry organ in these terms. There is one thing to remember that the brain is an organ so it cannot directly run on fat; it can only run on glucose or ketones. However, it becomes a necessary function for the brain to switch to ketones for survival. You might be surprised to know that fasting can achieve ketosis the quickest way, but apparently, that is not possible; therefore, the most efficient way for it is a ketogenic diet.

An average person's diet contains about 55% carbohydrates, 30% fat and 15% protein. When a person shifts to a keto diet, he/she eats more of fats and less of carbs, therefore 80% of the food comprises fat, about 15% of it is protein, and just 5% of calories come from carbohydrates. You should keep in mind that the preferred source of energy of our body is carbohydrates, so it always turns to use them first. However, if you eat few carbs, your body will finish them fast and will be forced to turn towards fats to break them down to get energy. This process can be beneficial for people who tend to lose a certain amount of weight, and it has so many other advantages than just this. A person can eat a strictly low-carb diet or a ketogenic diet for any amount of time.

Several advantages exist around a keto diet, ranging from therapeutic medical applications, weight loss to increased energy levels, etc. To make you more aware, here is a list of a few ways in which a keto diet can help you adopt a healthier lifestyle:

- **Weight loss:**

There are bodyweight loss benefits as your body fat is being used as a source of energy by being on a ketogenic diet. With its help, you alter your body into a machine that burns body fat as your insulin levels drop on a keto diet. It has also been scientifically proven that a ketogenic diet has shown better results regarding weight loss than high carb and a low-fat diet, even when we talk about long-term.

- **Controls body sugar:**

Because of the consumption of various food types, keto lowers your blood sugar levels naturally. One can also find in various researches that the keto diet is a more effective method to control and prevent diabetes, as compared to a low-calorie diet. One should seriously consider a ketogenic diet if you are diagnosed with Type II diabetes or also in case you are pre-diabetic.

- **Mental focus:**

After being on a ketogenic diet for some time, some people

noticed that it improved their mental focus and performance. It might be a little surprising to know that many people individually start a keto diet to increase or enhance their mental performance. You are not worrying about the unregulated spikes in the blood sugar while taking low carbs; therefore, ketones become fuel for the brain. This activity results in better concentration and an improved focus.

- **Better energy leading to normalized hunger:**

You feel the development of more energy in you when you give a reliable source of energy to your body. Fats have been shown to be the most active molecules, which can burn as fuel. In addition to that, it is already known that fats are more satisfying and leave you feeling full or satiated for a long time. This action helps you to cure your hunger pangs.

- **A cure for epilepsy:**

You might be amazed to know that the ketogenic diet has been used since the 1900's to cure epilepsy. It helps in offering excellent control, along with requiring fewer medications. It is one of the most preferred therapies for children who are still suffering from uncontrolled epilepsy. Not just children as recent studies have shown that the keto diet has been successful in treating adult epilepsy patients as well.

- **Blood pressure and cholesterol:**

A keto diet also improves cholesterol triglyceride levels that are associated with arterial build-up, as shown by studies. It leads to a significant increase in HDL and a decrease in LDL particle concentration in comparison to low-fat diets. Various studies also show that there has been an improvement in blood pressure levels being on a keto diet.

- **Insulin resistance:**

There are ample researches that show that a keto diet lowers the insulin levels in your body and brings them into a healthy range. It is also to be noted that if insulin resistance is left unattended, it can also lead to Type II diabetes. When you eat food high in omega three fatty acids, it can help you benefit from insulin optimization.

- **Acne reduction:**

When you switch to a keto diet, you will automatically observe some improvements in your skin. A study shows drops in skin inflammation and lesions when one turns to a low-carb diet. Another research shows a relation between consuming a high-carb diet and increased acne.

Chapter 3: Risks of a Keto Diet

Critical situations in which a keto diet might not work for you

Although a ketogenic diet has many benefits, it might not work for you in certain conditions or has some risks listed below.

- **Physical performance:** It is often argued that the keto diet affects your physical performance; however, it is not right in the end. You might have some side effects of it in the short run, such as one may notice a drop or a low in their physical performance, although it will subside when you continue to take fluids that replenish you, such as electrolytes. To fight this myth, researchers conducted a study on trained cyclists who had been on a keto diet for about four weeks. It was proven that aerobic endurance was not compromised at all along with their muscle mass still being the same as they had started. It was noted that their bodies had become familiar with ketosis, therefore limiting the glucose and glycogen stores and used fats as the predominant source of energy. One more study was conducted on eight professional gymnasts who eventually showed the same result. Both groups had been given a strict diet of proteins, green vegetables, and high-quality fats; however, the keto diet can give you a performance loss in exercises where one needs explosive action. In that case, if you need a boost in your performance, you can increase your carb intake by eating 25-30g of carbs, 30 minutes before training.

- **Ketoacidosis:** When the ketone production in your body gets too high, it is termed as ketoacidosis; however, it usually does not happen under normal circumstances. Often, for most people, it becomes a task to get into optimal ranges for ketosis. There are many misconceptions about the low carb diet. Thus, many skeptics are doubtful about the results of this diet plan. There have also been cases where people got confused with high fat and high card diets, which are not suitable for the body. It is not going to be good if you eat many fatty foods which are high in sugar, but it has been shown that a keto diet is healthier and more effective than low-fat dieting. As a caution, you must always check and discuss with your physician in case you have any concerns or queries about starting a keto diet.

- **Headaches and dizziness:** In the initial week, many people report problems, aggravation, dizziness and mental fogginess. Usually, it is the result of the electrolytes being flushed out of your body. Ketosis has a diuretic effect; therefore, to fight back these symptoms, it is essential for you to drink a fair amount of water and keep your sodium intake under control. It will help you replenish and feel better.

Chapter 4: What to Eat on a Keto Diet?

Easy ways to bring a change in your diet plan

Once you have decided that you want to start a keto diet, it is necessary to have a plan. One can enter ketosis as fast as they eat carbohydrates. One needs to keep the carbs very low in the diet. You can keep it limited from vegetables, dairy, and nuts. You are not supposed to eat any refined carbs, such as wheat in the form of bread, cereals, pasta; starch as in legumes, potatoes, beans or fruit. However, there are some fruits, which can be consumed in moderation, such as berries, avocado, and star fruit.

Do not eat:

- Fruits – oranges, apples, bananas, etc.

- Grains – wheat, cereal, corn, rice, etc.

- Tubers – yams, potatoes, etc.

- Sugars – maple syrup, honey, agave, etc.

Do eat:

- Avocados and berries – blackberries, raspberries, etc.

- High dairy fat – butter, hard cheese, high-fat cream, etc.

- Meats – beef, eggs, fish, poultry, lamb, etc.

- Sweeteners – monk fruit, stevia, erythritol, etc.

- Seeds and nuts – sunflower seeds, macadamias, walnuts, etc.

- Leafy greens – kale, spinach, etc.

- Above ground vegetables – cauliflower, broccoli, etc.

- Other fats – saturated fats, coconut oil, high-fat salad dressing, etc.

It must not be forgotten that a keto diet is extremely low in carbs, moderate in proteins, and high in fat. The ideal nutrient intake while being on a keto diet should be 5% carbohydrates, 25% proteins, and 70% fats. With low sugar intake, the overall results of your diet will be better. 20-30g net carbs are recommended for the keto diet. If you aim to lose weight through a keto diet, it will be good to keep track of your intake of net carbs and total carbs. In case you are wondering what precisely net carbs are, they are your total dietary carbohydrates minus the total fiber intake.

Vegetables to Eat on a Keto Diet:

Leafy and dark green vegetables seem to be the perfect choice for people on a keto diet. Your meals should have an extra side of fat along with proteins and vegetables. You can opt for chicken breasts in olive oil, with cheese and broccoli. Steak with a lot of butter and spinach sautéed in olive oil can also be a fantastic option.

Vegetable	Amount	Net Carbs
Cauliflower (steamed)	½ cup	0.9
Green beans (cooked)	½ cup	2.9
Broccoli (florets)	½ cup	2
Cabbage (green raw)	½ cup	1.1
Bok choi (Raw)	½ cup	0.2
Lettuce (Romaine)	½ cup	0.2
Kale (Steamed)	½ cup	2.1

There are 6g carbohydrates and 2g fiber in 1 cup.

Chapter 5: Sample Meal Plan

Sample meal plan for a week to start

Most of the time it gets difficult for people to figure out from where to start after making a decision that they want to be on a ketogenic diet. To help you with the same, here is a sample diet plan, which will help you in achieving your goals.

Monday

> → Breakfast: Tomatoes, bacon, and egg
>
> → Lunch: Chicken salad with feta cheese and olive oil
>
> → Dinner: Salmon, along with asparagus (to be cooked in butter)

Tuesday

> → Breakfast: Basil, egg, goat cheese omelet and tomato
>
> → Lunch: Cocoa powder, almond milk, stevia milkshake and peanut butter
>
> → Dinner: Cheddar cheese, along with vegetables and meatballs

Wednesday

> → Breakfast: Milkshake (it has to be ketogenic)
>
> → Lunch: Shrimp salad, along with avocado and olive oil
>
> → Dinner: Salad, pork chops, along with parmesan cheese

and broccoli

Thursday

- → Breakfast: Omelet along with onion, salsa, spices, peppers, and avocado

- → Lunch: Celery sticks and some nuts with guacamole and salsa

- → Dinner: Chicken served with pesto and stuffed cream cheese, along with vegetables low in starch and sugar

Friday

- → Breakfast: Cocoa powder, yogurt (free of sugar), along with peanut butter and stevia

- → Lunch: Beef cooked in coconut oil, along with vegetables

- → Dinner: A burger without the bun, with cheese, egg, and bacon

Saturday

- → Breakfast: A cheese and ham omelet, along with plants

- → Lunch: Slices of cheese and ham, along with nuts

- → Dinner: Spinach cooked in olive oil, white fish, and egg

Sunday

- → Breakfast: Fried eggs, along with mushrooms and bacon

→ Lunch: A burger with guacamole, salsa, and cheese

→ Dinner: Salad with eggs and steak

This plan can be of great use to you. It can provide you with the much-needed inspiration to start being on a healthy diet and work for the goals that you must have decided.

Tips for Eating Out on a Ketogenic Diet

Most of us might eat out during the week because of some party or celebration. On occasions like this, you might think that it would not be possible for you to carry on with the keto diet that you have started; however, it is not difficult. You can make the restaurant meals keto-friendly by choosing some easy and necessary steps. For example, most restaurants offer meat-based or fish-based dishes. You can order this and replace any food high in carbs with extra vegetables. Apart from this, meals based on egg would also prove to be an excellent option for you, such as an omelet or eggs and bacon. You can also give a twist to your burgers by making it bun-less. You can skip the bun, and your fries can be swapped with vegetables. You can also add extra eggs, avocado, bacon or cheese. If you go to a Mexican restaurant, one can enjoy a meal with any meat, along with cheese, sour cream, salsa, and guacamole. When we think of dessert, there is no need for one to feel disheartened as you can have it by asking for berries and double cream or a mixed cheese board.

Chapter 6: The Ways of Reaching Ketosis

Reaching ketosis requires a few specific ways to it

Reaching ketosis is not a difficult thing to do. It is a simple process. Find the following steps you need to enter that state:

1. **Restrict your carbohydrates:** The mistake most people do is that they only focus on net carbs. It is better to focus on net carbs and the total carbs intake of yours. Your net carbs should be below 20g, and total carbs should be around 35g a day.

2. **Control your protein intake:** It is essential for you to understand that along with your carbohydrates, protein intake is to be controlled too. When you take so many proteins, it might lower the levels of ketosis. If your main aim is to lose weight through a keto diet, then your protein intake should be between 0.6g and 0.8g per day.

3. **Do not worry about the fat:** It is typical of you to worry about the fat intake in a keto diet; however, you must not forget that fat is the primary source of energy in ketosis. You cannot lose weight through a keto diet by starving. You require the consumption of an ample amount of fat to see results.

4. **Drink water in abundance:** It is crucial to ensure proper hydration for your body. You must stay consistent with the amount of water you drink. One must try to drink a gallon of water every day. When you

drink enough water, it helps you control your hunger levels, along with regulating vital bodily functions.

5. **Avoid the habit of snacking:** It is not healthy to indulge in snacks. You will lose weight more efficiently when you have lesser insulin spikes during the day. Snacking will slow down the process of your weight loss.

6. **Add exercise to your schedule:** It may sound clichéd but exercising does many good. You must think of adding 20-30 minutes of activity in your plan, along with the keto diet to see differentiated results. It is okay to not indulge in a hardcore workout instantly, but even simple walks can do it for you. They can regulate your blood sugar levels and weight loss.

Chapter 7: Measuring Ketosis

Ways to measure ketosis

There are three ways to measure ketosis which come with their pros and cons, and are listed below:

- ❖ **Urine strips:** Using urine strips to measure ketosis is one of the simplest and the cheapest way to do so. It is an excellent option for beginners. The fundamental approach on how to use it is to dip the strip in your urine and, after fifteen seconds, the color of the piece changes to show the presence of ketones in your body. If you get a high reading, which is usually a dark purple color, you would automatically know that you are in ketosis. Its advantages count that it is readily available in pharmacies and is very cheap. It is a reliable test, which proves whether you are in ketosis, or not. However, the problem is that results can differ to a significant degree depending on the amount of fluid you drink. The strips are unable to show a precise ketone level. Once a person becomes keto-adapted, his/her body starts reabsorbing ketones from the urine, which would make urine stripes unreliable, even when you are in ketosis. The test can also show negative results when you have been in ketosis for several weeks.

- ❖ **Breath ketone analyzers:** Using breath-tone analyzers can be a simple way of measuring your ketones in your breath. They are more expensive than urine strips, but cheaper than blood ketone meters in the long run. These are re-useable for many times.

These analyzers, which not only give you the precise levels of ketones present in your body, they also provide a color code for a generic ketone level. What is interesting is that you can get your results via their app by hooking it up to a mobile phone or a computer and get an exact number of the ketones present. Various researches have shown that this device provides a decent correlation with the blood ketones in most cases. Its cons include that it might not always be accurate, along with being a little more expensive. They can show misleading values in some cases, and do not relate well with the ketones, although its re-usability and simplicity make it worth it.

❖ **Blood ketone meters:** Blood ketone meters remain successful in providing the exact value of ketones in your body. They are currently the most accurate way to show the ketone levels in one's body. They are the gold standard; but they are costly. Its reviews have been positive, and it has helped in knowing the exact amount of ketosis. It is precise and reliable, and its only con is that even, at present, it remains costly.

Chapter 8: Optimal Ketosis and Macros

Ways to know you are in ketosis

There are no specific ways to reach optimal ketosis. Dietary nutrition can accomplish it. It is just essential for you to remain vigilant and stay strict.

Ways to know if you are in ketosis:

There are a variety of ways by which you can see if you are in ketosis. One of them can be using urine strips, but they are not worth it because they might not be precisely accurate, along with being a little expensive; therefore, you can use the following 'physical symptoms,' which will let you know if you are on the right track:

- **Increased urination:** A keto diet causes an increased passing of urine, so you naturally have to go to the bathroom more. Acetoacetate, which is a ketone body, is excreted in the urination. Beginners might take time to adjust to the increased bathroom visits.

- **Increased thirst:** The increased urination leaves you with a dry mouth and increases appetite; therefore, it is imperative for you to drink plenty of water and stay hydrated. You must replenish your electrolytes.

- **Bad breath:** This is a temporary effect and goes away long-term. It happens due to acetone, which is a ketone body that is partially excreted in our breath. It can smell similar to nail polish remover or like over-ripe fruit.

- **Increased energy and reduced hunger:** One experiences a much lower hunger level after getting past the 'keto flu.' Along with this, you will also experience a clear or energized mental state.

One should not focus too much on testing and experimenting; instead, it is better to focus on your nutritional aspect. Your focus should be to take proper food and stay within your macro ranges. "Macro" is an abbreviation of the term 'Macronutrients.' Macros constitute of a daily intake of "the big 3" nutrients: carbohydrates, protein, and fats.

Chapter 9: Calculating Your Macros for Keto

Ways to calculate macros

The most important aspect of starting on the path of a ketogenic diet is getting your macros correct. It is crucial during the first weeks of a keto diet to track your macros, although sometimes it can be cumbersome. Tracking your macros gives you the essential feedback. Keto can bring a massive change. If you are a person coming from a standard American diet (SAD) background, your carbs will lower, the protein may go up or down, and fat will go up. If you are a person who is coming from the bodybuilding style diet, your levels of fat intake will increase tremendously and, most likely, your protein will drop. The macros end up looking like the following for most people:

- ✓ Carbohydrates: 5 to 9%

- ✓ Fats: 70 to 75%

- ✓ Proteins: 15 to 20%

Are you wondering from when you should start your calculations? You must start it with proteins and carbs. When you start the first round, it is good to keep your carbohydrate intake less than 50 grams per day. It is recommended to track net carbs by subtracting fiber from total carbs. For example, an avocado in total has about 12 grams of carbs but 10 grams of fiber; therefore, it has 10 grams of net carbs. One is advised to eat as many leafy vegetables as possible as they contain a lot of fiber. When it comes to the protein requirements of athletes, it should ideally range from 0.6 to 1.0g per lb. of lean mass and not per pound of bodyweight. There is an example below of how you can calculate the protein needs of a 180-pound lifter who has 20% body fat:

- 180 lbs. * 0.20 = 36 lbs. of fat

- 180 lbs. – 36 lbs. = 144 lbs. of lean mass

- 144 lbs. * 0.6 g = 86.4 g

- 144 lbs. * 1.0 g = 144 g

- Protein range = 87 – 144 g per day

Where, g = grams; lbs. = pounds

Chapter 10: Types of Ketogenic Diets

Achieve your goal with a suitable kind of keto diet for you

A keto diet is beneficial for the ones who want to build some muscle, although protein intake matters here. If one aims to gain mass, then the recommended protein intake is 1.0 - 1.2g per lean pound of body mass. If one wants to put on body fat, then it can be easy for you to achieve your goals by following the different types of ketogenic diets:

- Standard ketogenic diet (SKD): Everyone knows about this usual ketogenic diet. It is about the 'bread and butter.' It can be the best version for the ones who have just started it. Under this diet plan, one needs to consume 20-50g of net carbs per day. The protein intake has to be moderate and the fat intake has to be high. Consumption of 30g of net carbohydrates will induce ketosis.

- Targeted ketogenic diet (TKD): In this diet plan, you eat SKD, but, along with that, you also consume a small amount of fast digesting carbs before a workout. This diet is ideal for the ones who want to maintain their exercise performance and for the individuals who know their limits well. This diet allows for the re-synthesis of glycogen without interrupting the process of ketosis. If this is the plan you are looking forward to adopting, then aim for 25-50g of net carbs or less, along with 30 minutes to an hour for exercise. This activity will help you in making the carb intake for the day.

- Cyclical ketogenic diet (CKD): This is for the contest goers and the bodybuilders. This diet plan is about giving one day a week to carb up and re-supply glycogen stores. This diet plan is like a cycle of days between eating low-carbs and high-carbs. You might eat a low-carb diet for several days and a day or two of eating foods rich in carbs will follow it. This phenomenon can be termed as 'carb loading.' The high carb days in this diet plan can last between 24-48 hours. This diet plan requires 50g of carbohydrates per day during the first phase and then about 450-600g of carbohydrates during the period of carb loading.

- High protein ketogenic diet (HPKD): This diet is somewhat similar to the standard ketogenic diet, but it has more protein. In this diet plan, the body gets to adapt to this state and tends to lose the minimum amount of muscle tissue. The body uses dietary fat along with body fat for energy when it is fed with proteins and fat. It leaves the majority of the protein intake for muscle repair; however, over-eating protein can be wrong, and it can keep you away from reaching your goals.

The Types of Keto <u>Diets</u> and Muscle Maintenance

Many people might fear losing muscle while being on a keto diet; however, there are some specific mechanisms which can contribute to muscle growth even when you are on a ketogenic diet. It is already known that the liver produces ketones when carbs are absent. These ketones comprise protein-sparing properties, which help in the prevention of muscle breakdown. There is a main ketone, beta-hydroxybutyrate (BHB), and it has shown to promote protein synthesis. Another factor that remains important in preventing muscle mass is adrenaline. When the blood sugar reserves are low, it sends a strong message for adrenal secretion. It has shown that adrenergic influences regulate skeletal muscle protein mass.

Our body transmits a signal to the adrenal gland when the blood glucose drops from the intake of low-carbs to release epinephrine. Muscle protein is affected by the influence of the adrenal gland due to their hormonal activity of inhibiting the breakdown of muscle. A high-protein ketogenic diet emphasizes high protein intake, as an adequate amount of protein is a crucial factor in maintaining the muscle mass.

The Best Type of Keto Diet for You

There cannot be any definite answer to what kind of diet can work for you. The old 'calories in vs calories out' rule is not entirely correct, but it is proper to only a limited extent. What this rule does not take into account is the type of weight you are losing and whether it is lean mass or body fat. One can find a number of other variables to be put into place rather than just agreeing to this simple rule which indicates that it does not matter what you eat, what matters is that you eat less than you expend. Although it is agreed that a calorie deficit will result in weight loss, however, some of the weight loss could be coming from the muscle. There is research that a keto diet requires only 15-25% of the intake to be protein, and muscle mass can be prevented even during a caloric deficit in ketosis.

If the question of choosing the best diet for yourself remains with you, then it is recommended to determine the standard ketogenic diet (SKD). It can be of extreme help in acquainting your body to the new diet plan, and make the transition easier. The standard ketogenic diet will help in the alteration of your metabolism even if you are an athlete. Once your ketone levels are high enough, one can think of 'carb loading.' However, you are not supposed to use the carb loading days as your cheat days when you have cravings for carbs. It can soon put you out of ketosis so it it has to be a well-informed decision.

Chapter 11: Keto Flu

A typical experience for people who have newly switched to keto

When people make a transition to keto, they experience some discomfort which includes fatigue, nausea, headache, cramps, etc. There are two primary reasons for it, which are as follows:

1. Keto being a diuretic: When one opts for a keto diet, there is more need to go to the washroom to urinate due to which you lose your electrolytes and water from your body. However, this can be overcome by drinking Powerade Zero or eating a bouillon cube along with increasing your water intake. The main thing is to replenish your deteriorated electrolytes.

2. It is the transition: Your body can process a high intake of carbs and a low intake of fats; however, to do this, our body needs to create a few enzymes. When you have just made the transition, your brain will take time to adjust to it. Due to this, one might experience nausea, headaches, and grogginess as the energy intake is low. If this problem persists, then you can gradually increase your carb intake.

You should be relieved of all symptoms of keto flu after replenishing your electrolytes and drinking a fair amount of water. For an average person who has just started the ketogenic diet, it is advisable to eat 25-30g of carbs a day and the whole adaptation process will take about four to five days. It is also advised to cut your carbs fewer than 15g within one week to make sure that you are on your way to ketosis although, if the problem of keto flu persists, then you must consult your physician at once. If you are a person who avidly goes to the gym, you might notice that you lost some endurance and strength. Seeing a temporary decrease in physical performance is typical, but once your body gets wholly adapted to the keto diet, then the ability of your body to fully utilize fat as its primary source of energy will increase.

Chapter 12: Common Side Effects on a Keto Diet

Principal side effects for the ones who have just started

It has already been discussed that people who start with a keto diet experience a few issues, which are usually related to either dehydration or a lack of micronutrients or vitamins so it is advised to drink a lot of water and eat foods with micronutrients. Some of the few highlighted issues are as follows:

- **Cramps:** It is common to experience pains when you are in the initial stages of the ketogenic diet. Individually, leg cramps are very common; however, it is a minor issue. It represents a sign where your body lacks something, especially magnesium concerning minerals. To combat this, you must eat salt in the right proportions in your food and drink many fluids.

- **Constipation:** The most fundamental cause of this illness is dehydration. The solution to it is to drink plenty of water, close to a gallon a day. You must also make sure that the vegetables you eat have a lot of fiber. You can get a decent amount of fiber intake from non-starchy vegetables. In a case when that does not work, one can try taking a probiotic or psyllium husk powder.

- **Heart palpitations:** Once you make a transition to the keto diet, it might be common for you to notice that your heart starts beating faster and harder. You do not need to worry about it. You should ensure that you are drinking plenty of fluids and eating enough salt. It will be very helpful in getting rid of the problem. If this problem persists, then try taking potassium supplements once a day.

Along with these, there are also some of the less common side effects of a keto diet, which are as follows:

- **Breastfeeding:** Many studies are going on the topic of breastfeeding while being on a keto diet. Although nothing can be concretely concluded, it has been said that ketogenic diets are healthy to do while breastfeeding. It is suggested that you take 30-50g extra carbs to help your body produce milk for breastfeeding. Maybe you will have to add extra calories. It has been explicitly defined that 300-500 calories worth of extra fat help in producing milk. If you need more advice on this, you can contact your professional medical expert.

- **Hair loss:** It has often been noticed that people start losing hair in the initial days of starting a keto, and if you are experiencing hair loss within five months of being on a keto diet, it is entirely reasonable and temporary. To combat this, you can take a multivitamin and carry on with what you usually do. Although it is one of the infrequent side effects of keto, it can be lowered or minimized by making sure that you are not restricting your calories too much and get a proper sleep of 8 hours a day.

- **Increased cholesterol:** It is often termed as a good thing. There are many studies which show that the cholesterol levels increase while being on a low-carb, ketogenic diet. There is an increase in your cholesterol level due to an increase in HDL (good cholesterol). It lowers your chances of heart disease. One more thing one can notice is an increase in triglyceride counts, but that is very uncommon in people who lose weight. Once your weight loss normalizes, such effects will subside. Also, there is a tiny percentage of people who experienced increased LDL cholesterol as well. These high levels are harder to test, although usually exceptional. The danger of LDL cholesterol comes from the size and density. These are shown to be very healthy on a keto diet.

- **Gallstones:** There have been various studies on the keto diet and gallstones. These studies have shown that most people either improved their gallstones or cured them entirely while being on a keto diet. The second side of the same coin explains that many people reported having discomfort when they start out on low-carbs initially. If you honestly stick to your diet, you can gradually feel an improvement. There have also been questioning from people asking if they can start a ketogenic diet after their gallbladder has been removed. The reply to such a query is a definite yes. You might want to increase your fat in a gradual manner, allowing your system to get used to it.

- **Indigestion:** When one switches to a keto diet, it helps in getting rid of heartburns and indigestion. In some cases, people experience increased attacks when they initially start the keto diet. If you are still experiencing problems, limiting the amount of fat you take would possibly be the best option. You can gradually increase the amount you receive per day over a two-week period.

- **Keto rash:** It has been reported that many people start to itch when they switch to the keto diet; however, there has been no reliable scientific explanation for this, although it is decidedly less frequent and only a handful of people have complained about it. It is most likely the irritation from the acetone, which is excreted in sweat. The cure to this can be to look for better absorbing clothes, along with showering after activities that cause perspiration. If you keep on experiencing this issue, you can consider changing your exercise plan or increase your intake of carbs.

Chapter 13: Customize Your Ketogenic Diet

Ways to diet according to your terms

If one wishes not to follow the ketogenic diet plans laid down, then forming a ketogenic diet plan for yourself will not be a big task. You can create a diet for yourself in the following easy steps:

1. Determine your ideal body weight: You need to contemplate on the appropriate weight for your body. It can be the weight at which you feel best about yourself, and you can calculate it using various calculators available online.

2. Establish your daily calorie requirement: It is crucial for you to establish your daily calorie requirements to maintain your ideal body weight. You can again use the calorie calculators available online along with your ideal weight and activity level to be able to determine the calorie value you should be consuming to maintain an average weight or body mass index (BMI).

3. Figure out the number of proteins, carbs, and fats to eat: You can figure out your total intake of fat, protein, and carbohydrates with the help of your ideal weight and daily caloric intake in gram and calorie measures.

Protein, Fat and Carb Requirements

→ Protein requirements: Usually, the protein intake should be between 1 gram and 1.5 grams per kilogram of lean body mass or ideal body weight. If you want to calculate the lean body mass, it can be calculated by subtracting fat weight from the total weight. This requirement equals the weight of just your bones and muscles. In case you do not know yours, you can use the ideal body weight.

→ Carbohydrate amounts: Your fundamental goal should stay under 60 grams of carbohydrates per day, and this can be an individual goal as well. In case you have a lot of muscle mass and exercise a lot, you can eat a little more and stay in ketosis. You need to limit your carbohydrates if you have diabetes, are insulin resistant or suffering from other metabolic issues. You can lower your carbohydrate intake to below 30 grams if losing weight is your goal.

→ Fat amounts: It is essential to increase your fats while being on a ketogenic diet, as this is what it is all about. You need to make your body utilize the fats you are consuming instead of being dependent on the glucose. The calories you get from consuming oils and fats make up the balance of the calories after you subtract proteins and carb calories.

Chapter 14: Health Conditions that a Keto Diet Benefits

Ways in which a ketogenic diet can be a cure for significant health conditions

Various researches have been done on the association of a ketogenic diet with some significant health conditions to see if it is beneficial. The results have been auspicious in the following health conditions:

- **Metabolic syndrome:** Metabolic syndrome is characterized by insulin resistance and is often referred to as prediabetes. You can be at the risk of prediabetes if you have a larger waistline, low HDL cholesterol, elevating blood sugar levels, along with elevated triglycerides. People with metabolic syndrome are at an increased risk of heart disease, diabetes and other disorders related to insulin resistance. Following a ketogenic diet can help you combat these symptoms of metabolic syndrome. Some of the essential benefits include lower blood pressure and sugar levels, along with better cholesterol values. A 12-week study was conducted on people with metabolic syndrome who were made to follow a ketogenic diet. The result was that they lost about 14% of their body fat with the help of it. A keto diet helped in decreasing the triglycerides by more than 50%, along with experiencing many other improvements.

- **Glycogen storage disease:** People who are

diagnosed with the glycogen storage disease lack one enzyme which helps in storing glucose as glycogen or breaking glycogen down into glucose. There is not just one but various types of glycogen storage diseases based on the enzyme, which is missing. Usually, this disease is diagnosed in childhood. There are not the same symptoms for each kind of glycogen storage disease, and they are different for each, although these may include fatigue, muscle cramps poor growth, low blood sugar and an enlarged liver. The patients of the disease are often advised to eat foods high in carbs at frequent intervals so that glucose is abundantly available to their body all the time. Research has suggested that the keto diet can help some people with some glycogen storage disease. GSD III, also known as Forbes-Cori disease, affects the muscles and the liver. Ketogenic can work as a relief for the same by providing ketones, which can be used as an alternate fuel to the body. GSD V, also known as McArdle Disease, affects the muscles due to which there is a limited ability for the patient to exercise. If one person diagnosed with GSD V followed a ketogenic diet for a year, he would experience a 3 to 10-fold increase in his/her exercise tolerance, as proven by studies.

♦ **Polycystic ovary syndrome (PCOS):** Polycystic ovary syndrome is a disease, which results in infertility and irregular menstruation marked by hormonal dysfunction. Many women diagnosed with polycystic ovary syndrome are obese, along with having insulin resistance. It becomes difficult for them to lose weight. They are also at an increased risk of being diagnosed with Type II diabetes. People who meet the criteria for metabolic syndrome have symptoms affecting their physical appearance. They may include increased acne and facial hair, along with other signs about the masculinity to higher testosterone levels. A study was conducted on eleven women with PCOS who had started following a ketogenic diet, and their weight loss had averaged by 12%. There was a decline in the fasting insulin level by 54%, and their reproductive hormones had improved. Two out of the eleven women who were suffering from infertility became pregnant.

♦ **Diabetes:** Reduction in blood sugar levels are experienced by people diagnosed with diabetes while being on a ketogenic diet. It is right in the case of both people diagnosed with "Type I" and "Type II" diabetes. Several researches speak of this issue, which show that a low-carb diet has been helpful in controlling the blood sugar levels and has provided other health benefits as well. Researchers conducted a 16-week study on 21 diabetic people, and they found out that 17 of them were able to decrease their dosage of diabetes medication after being on a ketogenic diet. On average, the participants had also lost about 19 pounds, and there had been a reduction in their triglycerides, blood pressure and waist size. There was another study which compared the ketogenic diet to a moderate carb diet, and people in the ketogenic group had noticed a 0.6% decrease HbA1c. 12% of the participants had achieved a HbA1c below 5.7%, which is often considered to be normal.

♦ **Some cancers:** One of the leading causes of death worldwide is cancer. There have been numerous studies to search for ways to cure cancer, and some of them have described that a ketogenic diet is helpful in some cases when coupled with initial treatments, such as chemotherapy, surgery, and radiation. Several researches carried out have noted that obesity, Type II diabetes and increased blood sugar levels have a link with breast cancer and other forms of it. They suggest that tumor growth can be prevented by restricting carbs to lower the insulin and blood sugar levels. Mice studies show that the ketogenic diet has been successful in reducing the progression of various types of cancers, including cancers that spread to the other body parts. Some of the experts say that a ketogenic diet might prove to be extremely helpful in the case of brain cancer. Studies have shown improvement in brain cancer, such as in glioblastoma multiform (GBM) which is the most common form of brain cancer due to the ketogenic diet. It was found that 6 out of 7 patients had given a modest response to an unrestricted calorie keto diet, which was coupled with an anti-cancer drug. Even if the keto diet has not made a real significant influence, it has been known to enhance the lives as well as the lifestyle of the cancer patients.

♦ **Autism:** Autism Spectrum Disorder (ASD) is a disease that creates problems in communication and social interaction, along with repetitive behavior in some of the cases. Usually, it is diagnosed in childhood and can be treated with the help of speech therapy along with many others. Research on young mice and rats shows that a keto diet can prove to be of great help improving the autism spectrum disorder patterns. Some of the features of autism are common with epilepsy. It has been shown by various researches that a keto diet reduced overstimulation of brain cells in mice models of autism. A study was also conducted on 30 children diagnosed with autism, and it was found out that 18 of them showed improvements in the symptoms of autism after being on a ketogenic diet for about six months. There was also another case study in which a young girl with autism had followed a dairy-free and gluten-free ketogenic diet for several years. As a result, she had experienced various improvements along with resolution of obesity, and a seventy-point increase in her IQ level.

♦ **Parkinson's disease:** This medical condition is a nervous system disorder due to which there are low levels of signaling molecule dopamine. There are several symptoms due to the lack of dopamine, such as impaired posture, tremor, stiffness, and difficulty in writing and walking. Being on a ketogenic diet releases some proactive effects on the brain and nervous system. Due to this, it is being explored as a potential therapy for Parkinson's disease. During the research when mice and rats with Parkinson's disease were fed with ketogenic diets, it had led to protection against nerve damage and increased energy production, along with improved motor function. In another study, seven people with Parkinson's disease followed a classic ketogenic diet. Five of them had averaged a 43% improvement in the symptoms after about four weeks.

♦ **Obesity:** Various studies have shown that ketogenic diets are far more useful for losing weight rather than low-fat diets or calorie-restricted diets. It provides other health improvements as well. A study was conducted on men for 24 weeks in which some men were fed a keto diet and the others with a low-fat diet, and it was observed that men who were on a ketogenic diet had lost twice as much weight as the ones who ate a low-fat diet. In addition to that, the keto diet helps in dropping the triglyceride levels and increasing the HDL cholesterol or good cholesterol. One of the incredible ability of a ketogenic diet is to reduce hunger, and, due to this, it works well for weight loss. It has been found that low carbs and calorie-restricted diets helped people to feel less hungry in comparison to standard calorie-restricted diets. A ketogenic diet has appetite-suppressing properties due to which people who were on a ketogenic diet consumed much less even when they were given a chance to eat anything they want. Obese men who started being on a ketogenic diet were less hungry, had taken much fewer calories and lost about 31% more weight than the moderate carb group.

♦ **GLUT1 deficiency syndrome:** Glucose transporter 1 (GLUT1) deficiency syndrome is a rare genetic disorder. It involves deficiency of a protein that helps to move blood sugar into the brain. Symptoms are seen shortly after birth and may include difficulty in movement, developmental delay and sometimes seizures. Ketones do not require this protein to cross the blood to the brain, unlike glucose, due to which it remains helpful in this deficiency syndrome. The ketogenic diet effectively provides the fuel to children's mind. Keto diet therapy also works to improve the symptoms of the GLUT1 deficiency syndrome. The researchers have noticed an improvement in the co-ordination of muscles and a decrease in seizure frequency along with an increase in concentration and alertness in the children on keto diets. A study was conducted in 10 children who were diagnosed with the GLUT1 deficiency syndrome and who followed the modified Atkins diet (MAD), and they had experienced improvements in seizures. After six months, three out of the six had become seizure free.

♦ **Traumatic brain injury:** Traumatic Brain Injury (TBI) is a result of a car accident or a fall in which the head would have struck the ground or a blow on the head. It can have extremely devastating effects on the memory, physical function, and personality. Injured brain cells have decidedly fewer chances of recovery unlike cells of the other body parts. This effect is due to the cause that the ability of the body to use sugar after the head trauma is impaired and some researches have shown that people suffering from a traumatic brain injury can benefit from a ketogenic diet. Studies on rats show that a Keto diet immediately after the brain injury helps in reducing the brain swelling, improve recovery process along with increasing motor function. However, there was just one catch, which was that these effects seemed more prominent in the young rats rather than the older ones. However, more controlled studies on humans are needed before reaching any conclusions.

♦ **Multiple sclerosis:** Multiple sclerosis is a nervous system disorder that damages the protective covering of the veins leading to issues with communication between the body and the brain. Its symptoms include problems with movements, memory, balance, vision, and numbness. It was found that a Keto diet suppressed inflammatory markers in a mouse model while researching multiple sclerosis. The reduced inflammation had its benefits, such as leading to improvements in physical function, learning, and memory. Multiple sclerosis reduces the ability of the cells to use sugar as the source of energy. In many types of researches, the potential of a ketogenic diet in assisting with energy production and repair of cell in the multiple sclerosis patients. A study was conducted on 48 people who were diagnosed with the multiple sclerosis syndrome and significant improvements were found in the cholesterol, quality of life scores and triglycerides for those who followed a ketogenic diet for several days.

♦ **Non-alcoholic fatty liver disease:** One of the most common liver diseases in the western world is the non-alcoholic fatty liver disease (NAFLD). It is linked to Type II diabetes, obesity, and metabolic syndrome and there has been substantial evidence that there have been improvements in the non-alcoholic fatty liver disease patients after being on a keto diet. A study was conducted in which 14 obese men with the non-alcoholic fatty liver disease, metabolic syndrome followed a keto diet for about 12 weeks, and the results were noted. It was seen that there had been a significant decrease in blood pressure, weight and liver enzymes. It might be awe-inspiring to know that about 93% of the men had a reduction in their liver fat and about 21% of them had achieved complete resolution of non-alcoholic fatty liver disease.

♦ **Alzheimer's disease:** Alzheimer's disease is termed as a progressive form of dementia and is characterized by plaques and tangles in the brain which impair memory. It shares features of both epilepsy and Type II diabetes, which include the inability of the mind to properly use glucose, seizures, and inflammation linked to insulin resistance. It has been shown with the help of animal studies that the keto diet is effective in improving co-ordination and balance. However, it does not affect the amyloid plaque, which is the hallmark of this disease. The symptoms of Alzheimer's disease can be reduced and improved with MCT oil or esters that can be helpful in increasing the ketone levels. One controlled study was done with 153 people with Alzheimer's disease who took a MCT compound. This group of people showed improvements in mental function after 45 to 90 days.

♦ **Migraine headaches:** Migraine headaches involve sensitivity to light, severe pain and nausea. Various studies have suggested that migraine symptoms improve in people who follow ketogenic diets. An investigation had reported about the reduction in pain medication and migraine frequency in people who had been on a keto diet for a month. There is an interesting case study of two sisters who had been following a cyclical ketogenic diet for weight loss, and, in return, their migraine headaches had disappeared by the fourth week but returned during the eighth week.

Chapter 15: Studies on Low-carbs and Low-fat Diets

Ending the debate on low-carbs and low-fat diets

There are never-ending debates on carbohydrates versus fats. Some people believe that due to the increased fat in the food there has been an increase in health problems, specifically heart diseases. However, in recent years, an increasing number of studies have challenged the low-fat diet. It is now believed that low-carb diets are a better way to deal with obesity than low-fat diets. Below are some of the researches and studies which compare the low-carb and low-fat diets. Most of the reviews have been conducted on people diagnosed with health problems such as obesity, Type II diabetes and metabolic syndrome. The primary outcomes have usually been weight loss along with other risk factors, such as triglycerides, cholesterol, HDL cholesterol, LDL cholesterol, and blood sugar levels.

> ➢ **Foster GD, et al. New England Journal of Medicine, 2003, a study conducted on a low-carb diet for obesity.**

The study was done on 63 individuals who were randomly distributed in two groups, which were the low-carb group and low-fat group. The low-fat group was restricted of calories. This study was done for about 12 months. It was noted that the low-carb group had lost more weight than the low-fat group. The low-carb group had lost 7.3% of their total body weight in comparison to the low-fat group that had lost 4.5% of their body weight. The differences were statistically crucial at three and six months but not at twelve months. Along with the bodyweight, the loss-carb group also had improvements in their triglyceride levels and HDL cholesterol; however, other biomarkers were the same in the other group as well.

> **Samaha FL, et al. New England Journal of Medicine, 2003, a study conducted to draw comparisons between a low-carb diet and low-fat diet in severe obesity.**

The study was conducted on a group of 132 people who were diagnosed with severe obesity, and the research randomly distributed them into two groups: the low-carb group, and the low-fat group. These people had a BMI of 43. Many of them had Type II diabetes or metabolic syndrome. The low-fat dieters were restricted of calories. This study lasted for six months. As a result, the low-carb group had lost an average of 5.8 kg; on the other hand, the low-fat group had managed to lose only 1.9 kg. The difference was significant statistically. There was a reduction as much as three times in the weight of the low-carb group than the low-fat group. Along with this, several other developments were also noted, such as the triglyceride levels had gone down by 38 mg/dL in the low-carb group in comparison to the 7 mg/dL in the low-fat group. Insulin sensitivity had also improved on the low-carb group and had got slightly worse in the low-fat group. The fasting blood glucose levels had gone down by 26 mg/dL in the low-carb group; but, on the other hand, it was only about 5 mg/dL in the low-fat group. Therefore, overall, the low-carb diet had yielded better benefits.

> **Sondike SB, et al. The Journal of Pediatrics, 2003. A study to judge the effects of a low-carb diet and cardiovascular risk factor in overweight adolescents.**

A study was conducted on 30 overweight adolescents who were randomly divided into two groups, which were the low-carb group and the low-fat group. The study had gone on for 12 weeks. Neither of the two groups was supposed to restrict calories as informed in the instructions. The results showed that the low carb group had lost 9.9 kg and, on the other hand, the low-fat group had lost about 4.1 kg. The weight loss was about 2.3% more in a low-carb group than the low-fat group. Along with this, significant decreases were also noticed in non-HDL cholesterol and triglycerides. Total and LDL cholesterol had decreased only in the low-fat group.

> ➢ **Brehm BJ, et al. The Journal of Clinical Endocrinology & Metabolism, 2003. A study comparing a low-carb diet and a calorie-restricted low-fat diet on cardiovascular risk factors and body weight in healthy women.**

The study was conducted n 53 healthy but obese women who were divided into the two groups, which were the low-carb group and the low-fat group. The low-fat group had been instructed on the restriction of calories. The study took place within 6 months. It was observed that the women in low-carb diet had lost an average of 8.5 kg, while the low-fat group women had lost 3.9 kg on average. The differences were significantly different by six months; therefore, the low-carb group had lost about 2.2 times as much as the low-fat group. Along with this, there had been reductions in blood triglycerides, and the HDL had improved in both the groups of women.

> ➢ **Aude YW, et al. Archives of International Medicine, 2004. The study conducted was to compare the National Cholesterol Education**

Program diet and a diet low in carbs and high in proteins and monounsaturated fat.

The study was conducted on 60 overweight individuals who were randomly distributed into two groups, one that was given a low-carb diet in monounsaturated fat and the other group was given a low-fat diet based on the National Cholesterol Education Program. The study was carried out for 12 weeks, and both groups were on a calorie-restricted diet. It was noticed that the low-carb group had lost about 6.2 kg on average, while the low-fat group had lost 3.4 kg in comparison. To conclude, the low-carb group has lost about 1.8 times of the weight as much as the low-fat group. Several significant changes showed up in the biomarkers, such as the waist-to-hip ratio had improved slightly in the low-carb group and not in the low-fat group. However, the total cholesterol had developed in both groups. The triglycerides had gone down by 42 MD/dL in the low-carb group as compared to 15.3 mg/dL in the low-fat group. The LDL particle size had increased by 4.8 nm and the percentage of small LDL had decreased by 6.1% in the low-carb group. However, there was no noticeable difference in the low-fat groups.

> ➢ **Yancy WS Jr, et al. Annals of Internal Medicine, 2004. The study conducted to compare the keto diet versus a low-fat diet to treat hyperlipidemia and obesity.**

The study was conducted on 120 overweight individuals who had increased blood lipids were categorized randomly into two groups, which were the low-carb group and the low-fat group. The calories were restricted for the low-fat group. The study took place over 24 months. It was noted that the low-carb group had lost about 9.4 kg on average in comparison to the low-fat group which lost 4.8 kg of their total body weight. The people of the low-carb group had also witnessed improvements in their HDL cholesterol and blood triglyceride levels.

> **JS Volek, et al. Nutrition and Metabolism (London), 2004. The study conducted was to compare an energy-restricted low-carb diet with the low-fat diet on body composition in overweight men and women and weight loss.**

The study was conducted on 28 obese individuals. The study had taken place for 30 days in the case of the women and 50 days for the men. Both the low-carb and low-fat diets were calorie-restricted. As a result, the low-carb group reduced more weight compared to the low-fat group, especially the group comprising of men. Thus, it concluded that way, even though they had eaten more calories than the low-fat group. The men on the low-carb diet have lost about three times as much weight of abdominal fat as the men on a low-fat diet.

> **Meckling KA, et al. The Journal of Clinical Endocrinology & Metabolism, 2004. The study conducted was to compare a low-fat diet to a low-carb diet on body composition, risk factors in cardiovascular disease in overweight men and women, and weight loss.**

The study was conducted on 40 overweight individuals who were randomly distributed in the low-carb and low-fat groups for ten weeks. The calories had to be matched between the two groups. In the result, it was noted that the low-carb group of people had lost some 7 kg, while the low-fat group had lost 6.8 kg. There was not much difference in their weights, and both of the groups had lost similar amounts. Although there were some noticeable differences in biomarkers, such as the blood pressure had reduced in both groups, systolic and diastolic, the total and LDL had also decreased in the low-carb group only. There was a decrease in triglycerides in both groups. There was an increase in HDL cholesterol in the low-carb group, but it had decreased in the low-fat group. Blood sugar had lowered in both groups, but only the low-carb people had a decrease in their insulin levels. This result was an indication of improved insulin sensitivity.

> **Nickols-Richardson SM, et al. Journal of The American Dietetic Association, 2005. A study was conducted on whether the perceived hunger and weight loss are more significant in obese premenopausal women who were on a low-carb/high-protein vs. high-carb/low-fat diet.**

The study was conducted on 28 premenopausal women who ate either a low-carb or low-fat diet for about six weeks. There was a restriction of calories for the low-fat group. It was noticed that women who were in the low-carb group had lost 6.4 kg weight in comparison to the group which consumed a low-fat diet as they had lost 4.2 kg. It was therefore concluded that the low-carb diet had proven to be more helpful in losing weight and reduced hunger when compared to the low-fat diet.

> **Daly ME, et al. Diabetic Medicine, 2006. The study conducted to know the short-term effects of severe dietary-restriction advice in Type II diabetes.**

The study was conducted on 102 people who were randomly distributed into two groups who were given low-carb and low-fat diets respectively for three months. The instruction of reducing the portion sizes was given to the low-fat group. At the end, it was noted that the low-carb group had lost 3.55 kg weight while, on the other hand, the low-fat group had lost only 0.92 kg. The difference was significant statistically. Along with the reduction in weight, it was also noticed that the low-carb group had seen more significant improvements in total cholesterol or HDL ratio; however, there was no difference in triglyceride levels, blood pressure or HbA1c between groups.

> ➢ **McCleron FJ, et al. Obesity (Silver Spring), 2007. A study conducted to know the effects of a low-carb keto diet and a low-fat diet on hunger, mood and other symptoms.**

The study was conducted on 119 overweight or obese individuals who were distributed into two groups at random, which were the low-carb keto group and the low-fat group. The research was done for six months. Results showed that the low-carb group had lost 12.9 kg of weight, whereas the low-fat group had only been able to lose 6.7 kg of weight. The people in the low-carb group had lost twice the weight as the people of the low-fat group, and they also experienced less hunger.

> ➢ **Gardner CD, et al. The Journal of The American Medical Association, 2007. Study on a comparison of Ornish, Atkins, Zone and LEARN diets for changes in weight and other risk factors among obese premenopausal women: The A to Z weight loss story.**

The research was conducted on 311 obese premenopausal

women who were randomly distributed into four groups which were given four different diets, such as a low-fat vegetarian Ornish diet, the LEARN diet, a low-carb Atkins diet and the Zone diet. The LEARN and Zone diets were calorie-restricted. The research was conducted for 12 months. It was found out that the Atkins group of women had lost the most weight in comparison to the other groups. They had lost 4.7 kg of weight in 12 months, and the Ornish lost 2.2 kg of mass, the LEARN lost 2.6 kg weight, and the Zone had lost about 1.6 kg weight. Nevertheless, the difference was not different statistically at 12 months. Along with the most significant weight loss by the Atkins group, they also had experienced improvements in HDL, blood pressure, and triglycerides. It was also noted that Ornish and LEARN had witnessed a decrease in LDL in 2 months, but then these effects diminished.

> **Halyburton AK, et al. American Journal of Clinical Nutrition, 2007. Study to know whether low and high-carb diets have similar effects on mood or cognitive performance.**

The study was conducted on 93 obese individuals who were randomly given to eat a low-carb, high-fat diet or low-fat, high-carb diet. This research was done for eight weeks. The calories for both the groups were restricted. It was noticed in the result that the low-carb group of people had lost 7.8 kg while, on the other hand, the low-fat group had lost 6.4 kg of weight. The difference was significant statistically. In the end, it was noted that both the groups had somewhat similar improvements in their mood, but the speed of processing was improved on the low-fat diet; however, the low-carb group lost more weight.

> **Dyson PA et al. Diabetic Medicine, 2007.**

Research on whether a low-carb diet is more effective in losing weight than healthy eating habits in both diabetic and non-diabetic people.

The research was conducted on 26 people; 13 were diabetic, and the other 13 were non-diabetic. They were randomly distributed into two groups who were supposed to eat a low-carb diet or a healthy eating diet which was according to the Diabetes UK recommendations. The study had taken place over three months. It was finally noticed that the low-carb group of people had lost 6.9 kg of weight, while the low-fat group of people had lost 2.1 kg of weight. The low-carb group had lost about three times weight as much as the low-fat group.

➢ **Westman EC, et al. Nutrition and Metabolism (London), 2008. The study conducted was to compare the effects of a low-carb ketogenic diet to a low-glycemic index diet on the glycemic control in Type II Diabetes Mellitus.**

The research was conducted on 84 individuals who were diagnosed with Type II diabetes and were obese as well. They were divided into two groups who were made to eat either a low-carb ketogenic diet or a low-glycemic diet which would be calorie- restricted. The study was completed in 24 weeks. In the end, it was noticed that the low-carb people had lost more weight in comparison to the low-glycemic group. The low-carb people had dropped 11.1 kg of body mass, while the low-glycemic people had lost about 6.9 kg. Other than the difference in weight, there was a change in other things as well, such as hemoglobin Ac1 had gone down by 1.5% in the low-carb group in comparison to the 0.5% in the low-glycemic look. The HDL cholesterol of only the low-carb group of people had increased too by 5.6 mg/dL. The diabetes medication of the people in the low-carb group could either be reduced or eliminated in 95.2%; on the other hand, only 62% was the reduction or elimination rate for the low-glycemic group. Blood pressure and triglycerides had improved in both groups; however, the differences between the groups had not been statistically significant.

> **Shai L, et al. New England Journal of Medicine, 2008. The study was conducted to compare weight loss with a low-carb diet, Mediterranean, low-fat diet.**

The research was conducted on 322 obese individuals who were randomly distributed into three groups who were made to follow three diets, which were a low-fat calorie restricted diet, a low-carb diet or a Mediterranean diet restricted in calories. The study took a time of 2 years. In the result, it was noted that the low-carb group had lost 4.7 kg of weight, the low-fat group had lost 2.9 kg, and the Mediterranean diet group had lost 4.4 kg weight. It was therefore concluded that the low-carb group of people had more influence than the other two groups and there also had been improvements in their triglycerides and HDL cholesterol.

> **Keogh JB, et al. American Journal of Clinical Nutrition, 2008. Research conducted to know the effects of weight loss from a low-carb diet on endothelial function and the markers on the cardiovascular disease risk about abdominal obesity.**

The research was conducted on 107 individuals who were diagnosed with abdominal obesity and were randomly distributed into a low-carb diet group and low-fat diet group. Both groups were calorie-restricted. The study took place in 8 weeks. It was eventually noticed that people from the low-carb group had lost 7.9% of their body weight, which was more in comparison to the low-fat group who had lost 6.5% of body weight; hence, the low-carb group of people had lost more weight. However, there was no difference in Flow Mediated Dilation or any other markers of the endothelium.

> **Tay J, et al. Journal of The American School of Cardiology, 2008. Research to know about the metabolic effects of weight loss in comparison to an isocaloric high-carb diet in abdominally overweight people.**

The study was conducted on 88 individuals who had been diagnosed with abdominal obesity. They were randomly distributed into two groups which had to consume a low-fat diet or a low-carb diet. The research was done over 24 weeks. Both the menus were supposed to be calorie-restricted. In the end, it was noted that the people of the low-carb group had lost 11.9 kg weight on average, while, on the other hand, people of the low-fat group had lost 10.1 kg which was lesser than the former. However, it was also noted that the triglycerides, insulin sensitivity, HDL, blood pressure and C reactive protein had improved in both groups, although total and LDL cholesterol had improved in the people of the low-fat group only.

> **Volek JS, et al. Lipids, 2009. Research conducted to know whether carb restriction has a more favorable impact on the metabolic syndrome than a low-fat diet.**

The study was done on a group of 40 people who had an increased risk of cardiovascular disease. They were randomly distributed into two groups who were supposed to eat a low-fat diet and a low-carb diet. The study was completed in 12 weeks. The calories were restricted for both groups. In the result, it was noticed that the low-carb group of people had lost 10.1 kg weight, while the low-fat group had lost 5.2 kg. The weight lost by the low-carb group was almost double compared to the loss by the low-fat group when both the groups ate the same amount of calories. Other than the weight, there were other things to be highlighted as well. The triglycerides had gone down by 107 mg/dL on a low-carb group, whereas it was only 36 mg/dL on the low-fat diet group. The result also showed an increase in the HDL cholesterol level by 4 mg/dL on the low-carb group, and it went down by only 1 mg/dL on the low-fat group. LDL size had increased on the low-carb group, but it had stayed the same on the low-fat group. Apolipoprotein B had also gone down by 11 points on the low-carb group, whereas it had only gone down by one spot on the low-fat group. The LDL particles had shifted partly from small to large, and, on the other hand, they had partially moved from large to short in the case of the low-fat group.

> **Brinkworth GD, et al. American Journal of Clinical Nutrition, 2009. A study conducted to know about the effects of a low-carb diet for weight loss in comparison to an isocaloric low-fat diet after 12 months.**

The research was conducted on 118 people who were diagnosed with abdominal obesity and were distributed into two groups at random in which they had to be on a low-fat diet or a low-carb diet. This research was done for one year. Both diets were restricted from calories. It was noticed that the low-carb group had lost about 14.5 kg of weight, whereas the low-fat group lost 11.5 kg; however, the difference was not significant statistically. It was noted that the low-carb group of people experienced a decrease in the triglycerides and an increase in both HDL and LDL cholesterol in comparison to the low-fat group.

> **Hernandez, et al. American Journal of Clinical Nutrition, 2010. Research on the lack of suppression of free fatty acids circulating and hypercholesterolemia during weight loss on a low-carb and high-fat diet.**

The research was conducted on 32 obese people who were distributed into two groups at random, the groups being a low-fat diet group and a low-carb group. It was carried out for six weeks. It was noticed that the low-carb group had lost 6.2 kg weight, while, on the other hand, the low-fat group of people had lost 6.0 kg weight on average. The difference was not significant statistically. Along with the weight loss, it was also noted that the low-carb group had experienced a decrease in triglycerides by 43.6 mg/dL, while the low-fat group had experienced it at 26.9 mg/dL; however, HDL and LDL had decreased in the low-fat group only.

> **Krebs NF, et al. Journal of Pediatrics, 2010. The study was on safety and efficacy of high protein, low-carb diet for weight loss in obese adolescents.**

The study was conducted on 46 people who were distributed into two groups at random to follow either a decreased carb diet or a low-fat diet. The research was completed in 36 weeks.

The low-fat group had calorie restrictions. In the result, it was noticed that the low-carb group had lost more weight and there was a much more significant decrease in BMI of the people in the low-carb group than the low-fat group. However, one could not find any significant differences between both groups.

> **Guldbrand, et al. Diabetologia, 2012. Research to see that in Type II diabetes, a low-carb diet is to be followed and how it improves glycaemic control in comparison with advice to follow a low-fat diet to have a similar weight loss.**

The study was conducted on 61 individuals who were diagnosed with Type II diabetes. They were distributed into two groups at random who had to follow either a low-fat diet or a low-carb diet. This study was to be done over two years. Both diets were supposed to be calorie-restricted. It was noted that the low-carb group of people had lost 3.1 kg, whereas the low-fat group lost 3.6 kg weight; however, the differences were not significant statistically. There was no difference in weight loss, but there was a substantial improvement in the glycemic control for six months for the people in the low-carb group, but the compliance was not good, and the effects had diminished within 24 months as the people had increased their carb intake.

Accomplishments:

It was seen that 21 out of 23 studies showed that low-carb groups had been more effective in losing weight. Some of the facts which must be noted are as follows:

- The low-carb groups lost 2-3 times more weight than

the low-fat groups. In other cases, there was no difference between the two.

- In most cases, the low-carb group of people could eat as many calories as they wanted, but the calories were restricted for the low-fat group.

- When the calories were restricted for both groups, the people who were on a low-carb diet lost more weight; however, it was not always significant.

- There was just one study which showed that the low-fat group had lost more weight than the low-carb group; however, the difference was minimal and not even significant statistically.

- When the researchers looked at the abdominal fat cases, they saw that low-carb groups were an advantage.

- The main reasons why low carbohydrate diets are so successful in losing weight are their appetite-suppressing effects, along with its high protein content. This effect automatically leads to a reduction in calorie intake.

- Despite concerns expressed by some people, low-carb diets do not raise LDL cholesterol levels on average. None of the studies have shown any real adverse effects.

- Low-carb diets raise HDL levels as more fat is eaten during the keto diet. Higher HDL is related to better and improved metabolic health and a lesser risk of cardiovascular diseases. Having low HDL is one of the symptoms of metabolic syndrome.

- The best way for one to reduce triglyceride levels is to eat fewer carbohydrates which automatically happens in a low-carb or keto diet; therefore, in the researches above, 19 out of 23 reported a change in the triglyceride levels.

- In people who were non-diabetic, insulin and blood sugar levels had improved on both low-fat and low-carb diets and the difference between them was undeniably less.

- Three studies compared low-fat and low-carb diets in the Type II diabetes patients. Only one of those studies had been able to reduce carbohydrates sufficiently. It was also noted that about 90% in the low-carb group had been able to eliminate the medications of diabetes; however, the difference was tiny in the other two studies as the compliance was very poor.

- Blood pressure was decreased on both low-carb and low-fat diets.

Chapter 16: Frequently Asked Questions (FAQ)

Answers to some of the common questions

Q: How much body mass will I decrease?

A: The amount of body mass that you lose depends on only one factor, and that is you. Although, if you add exercise to your schedule, you are going to lose much more weight at a faster pace. For this, you must cut out some foods from your diet, such as weight products, artificial sweeteners, dairy products, etc.

Water weight loss is not uncommon in a keto diet. A keto diet has a diuretic effect to it, due to which you lose many pounds in just some days. However, it is not fat mainly; it only means that your body is trying to adjust itself to the new changes that have been brought, and how it has to work as a fat burning machine.

Q: How will I be able to track my carb intake?

A: There are various mobile apps which can help you to a great length in tracking your carb intake along with fiber intake. You can complete this by yourself by calculating net carbs. They can be calculated by subtracting your total fiber intake from the total carb intake.

Q: I cheated on my diet and wanted to get back on it. How do I do it?

A: It is not something heinous. It is probably okay to cheat sometimes; however, as a consequence of this, your bodyweight will temporarily go up as your body will start retaining water. You will figure out that you will automatically lose weight when your body starts releasing the stored water although, if you plan to get back to the diet, it is essential for you to buck up and get back on track. You should remain strict if you have cravings.

Q: I have stopped losing weight. Now what?

A: You might now know, but there are various factors which might be slowing your weight loss process unknowingly, such as hormonal changes, lack of sleep, exercise, stress, and alcohol use. Also, you must know that weight loss cannot be a linear process. There are fluctuations in water retention or water release every day. People usually lose 1-2 lbs on average, but this does not give a guarantee that the scale is going to drop consistently. You must start looking at your dietary choices if you are having problems after 4-5 weeks of being on a ketogenic diet.

The first recommendation is to re-check your macros and make sure that they have been on track.

Q: I do not like eggs/dairy/meat, so is it still possible for me to do a ketogenic diet?

A: You can consider a yes as an answer to this query. There are no specific written down rules to do a ketogenic diet except for maintaining low carbs, moderate proteins, and high fats. If you are not comfortable with eating eggs, dairy or meat, then you opt for some vegetarian recipes available online. Some people also drink coffee with butter. There are plenty of options available even if you are looking for a vegetarian meal.

Q: What will happen once I reach my goal weight on keto?

A: It remains a personal choice of being on keto or not after reaching your ideal weight. Some people choose to get off the diet, while some continue it or try to stay on a clean-eating diet. The only principle you need to remember is to not go back to your old habits as you would tend to gain weight by doing so.

Q: Can I eat carbs ever again?

A: If you are in the initial stages of your diet, it is advised for you to eliminate them, although, after being on a diet for 3-4 months, you can eat carbs but only on special occasions, and to return to your diet plan immediately after it.

Q: Am I going to lose muscle while being on a keto diet?

A: It is accepted that there is some risk of losing muscle on a keto diet; however, you can try to minimize your muscle loss by keeping your protein intake high along with high ketone levels.

Q: What if I continuously feel fatigued and tired all the time?

A: If you tend to feel tired all the time, it is possible that you might not be efficiently utilizing your ketones and fats. You can effectively combat this by lowering your carb intake.

Q: Is there any exact amount of protein to be taken on a ketogenic diet?

A: The ketogenic diet is based on the principle of moderate proteins. If you keep your protein intake very high, it can cause an increase in your insulin levels along with lowering your ketones. The upper limit for it is 35% of the total calorie intake.

Conclusion

It has been proven by various researches and studies how effective a ketogenic diet is and all the good it does to the body, from curing diseases to providing multiple other health benefits. The ketogenic diet has become a kind of revolution and can help in changing the lives of people in a healthier and happier way.

There are many benefits of a ketogenic diet. It increases the complete development of the mind and body, and therefore it helps in increasing mental focus and concentration. It also works wonders in reducing the medication of so many diseases or disorders. What could be more spectacular than being helpful in improving the health of cancer patients? It is a diet which should be recommended to everyone to at least try once and notice the differences on their own.

Although a keto diet has its risks, most of them are short-term. It is all about transforming to the process of ketosis, and once your ketones start getting used efficiently you notice that all those risks or cons of the keto diet vanish on their own. Recently, there has been another exciting research which says that being on a ketogenic diet can help us live longer; thus, we can conclude that it has a robust effect on the people who are on this diet. The ketogenic diet has been known to boost metabolism and improves mental health. Another research tells that a ketogenic diet also helps to cure anxiety. It leaves a soothing effect on people who are suffering from anxiety but are making efforts to be on a ketogenic diet. There are countless studies about all the good that a keto diet has to offer.

There are uncountable success stories of people who have been on a ketogenic diet and reached their desired weight and, not just that, it has also helped in making them happier and improving their moods. There are many other diets available as well, but there are ample researches which have proven that it is better than most of them. Many types of studies have been discussed which demonstrate that a diet low on carbohydrates is so much better than a diet low on fats; hence, one must try a ketogenic diet to move towards a healthier lifestyle.

Bonus!

Wouldn't it be to know when Amazon's top kindle books go on Free Promotion? Well now is your chance!

I would like to give you full access to an exclusive service that will email you notifications when Amazon' top Kindle books go on Free Promotion. If you are someone who is interested in saving a ton of money, then simply go to the link below for Free access.

https://bit.ly/2xFpfOX

As a "Thank you" for downloading this book, I would like to give you "30 Day Low Carb Diet Ketosis Plan" ebook.

References

All the websites that have been referred

https://www.healthline.com/nutrition/23-studies-on-low-carb-and-low-fat-diets#section2

https://www.healthline.com/nutrition/15-conditions-benefit-ketogenic-diet#section16

https://www.healthline.com/nutrition/ketogenic-diet-101#section14

https://www.ruled.me/guide-keto-diet/#dangers-of-keto

https://www.healthline.com/nutrition/low-carb-diets-and-performance#section6

https://www.dietdoctor.com/low-carb/dining-out

https://www.dietdoctor.com/low-carb/ketosis

https://www.dietdoctor.com/low-carb/with-diabetes-medications

https://www.dietdoctor.com/low-carb/keto

https://www.healthline.com/health-news/keto-diet-can-help-you-live-longer-researchers-say#5

The Complete Beginner's Guide to Dairy Free Keto

direct or indirect, which are incurred as a result of the use of information contained within this document, including, but not limited to, —errors, omissions, or inaccuracies.

Introduction

First of all, I would love to thank you purchasing this book' *Dairy Free keto cookbook'!* I hope you find it is interesting and that it helps you with the keto diet.

We live in a day and age when there is a lot of focus on staying fit and leading a healthy lifestyle. It is more than just a personal aim to constantly maintain being at our fittest, whether we are 17 or 70!

Everyone has their own reason as to why they want to go on a diet – it could be anything from weight loss to an overall fit lifestyle. But then they are obstructed by doubts – is it worth it to give up on the foods they love?

Well, fret not! This book has been crafted especially for your needs and to remove whatever doubts you might be having. Contained within the chapters, you will find ample amounts of information detailing what the ketogenic diet is and how you can benefit from it, along with why dairy-free is such a good idea.

This diet, along with its dairy-free aspect, has gained immense popularity and all for the right reasons. It is recommended by experts all around the world because of the innumerable ways the human body benefits from it. Apart from all the valuable information, you will also find dairy-free keto recipes that will catapult you into your dairy-free keto journey.

Thank you once again for choosing this book.

Chapter One: The Ketogenic Diet

The Ketogenic diet in its simplest definition is a diet that has low carbohydrate content and, in contrast, a much higher content of fat. It is also commonly referred to as the LCHF diet - low carb, high fat.

In the keto diet, the dietary expectation of you is to make sure your intake of protein rich foods is appropriate, as this is the very foundation of the diet. There was a time when it was used as a treatment method for many types of ailments and diseases, whereas currently, it has garnered vast amounts of popularity for its effectiveness in weight loss, especially for those who are taking up the keto diet specifically to lose weight.

All around the world, it is being hailed by experts and specialists as the diet that can change your life with the smallest of alterations made in your dietary habits and lifestyle.

Normally, what happens in your body is that it burns carbohydrates in order to generate energy for you to function on. While on the keto diet, fats do the job of being the primary source of energy. Any person with a normal diet ends up consuming enormous quantities of carbohydrates, be it as a choice or something they consider to be the general approach to diets. But it is important to note that when carbohydrates are converted into glucose, the vast amounts of carbs turn into outrageous amounts of glucose that are released into your bloodstream, which in turn leads to weight gain.

This is where the ketogenic diet steps in. The replacement of carbohydrates with fats turns them into ketones. And in turn – ketones become the principal energy source. You will read about the innumerous health benefits of the ketogenic diet in the upcoming segments of this book.

Keto and its Types

There isn't just one – there are many types of ketogenic diets. Some of the common forms are:

- **High-Protein Ketogenic Diet:** In this diet, the protein quantity dominates the rest of the components of the diet.

- **Targeted Ketogenic Diet (TKD):** Here you are permitted to include carbohydrates in the diet with the condition that you engage in an intense and regular workout regime.

- **Standard Ketogenic Diet (SKD):** This diet's standard meal is supposed to consist of 5% carbs, 75% fat, and 20% proteins.

- **Cyclical Ketogenic Diet (CKD):** Intake days that are high in carbohydrates are allowed.

Chapter Two: Ketosis and the Science behind It

Ketosis

Our body sources its energy from glucose. Glucose is a form of sugar that is produced by sugars and dietary carbohydrates. These include:

- Sugar: foods like fruit and dairy
- Anything high in starch: noodles, rice, wheat and fries, etc.

Upon consumption, your body breaks down the carbohydrates into simple sugars. This is also the category of sugars glucose belongs to, and it is instantly used as fuel for your body. Either that, or it stores up in the liver, and that stored up glucose is a chemical that is known as glycogen.

When the generated amount of glucose falls short to meet your body's need for energy, the body shifts its focus to sourcing the required energy from other ways. One of the main methods includes the breakdown of fat stored in the body and assembling glucose straight from triglycerides. This way of functioning of our body leads to the release ketones. And the process of releasing ketones is called ketosis.

Ketones

Ketones are a type of acid. They accumulate in your body as it goes through the process of ketosis.

They act as a sign of the successful breaking down of fats and the body entering ketosis.

But it is worthy to note that ketones in excess amounts could impact your body in a negative manner and result in a condition known as ketoacidosis.

To Enter Ketosis

Reaching ketosis is not a difficult process although, it might get very confusing for most people, as there is a lot of information on this matter. Here's how ketosis can be attained properly.

Your consumption of carbohydrates being restricted is the most essential aspect of attaining ketosis. In fact, it is also the most vital factor of the keto diet itself. Here, there are two things to be kept in mind:

- Focus on the total carbs
- Focus on the net carbs

The goal is to stay below 35 g of total carbs and 20g of net carbs, per day.

A restriction on your intake of protein is also just as important as restricting your carb intake.

Contrary to the misconception of a lot of people, a high consumption of protein is not necessary as that could lead to weakening the impacts of ketosis. In order to keep a daily check and track of your nutrient levels, consider using ketogenic diet calculators.

Some Important Points to Note:

- Working out helps amplify whatever effects the keto diet could have on your body.
- Fast over starve – fasting can be an effective tool when it comes to spike up your ketone levels and helps keep them engaged all day long.
- Stay hydrated no matter what. You should drink at least a gallon of water on a daily basis. A gallon should be the minimum! Not only that, but drinking water helps in controlling hunger levels as well,
- Consume the required supplements – when you are on a keto diet, if you feel any kind of weakness in your body, it is advisable you consider opting for vitamins, minerals, etc. supplements.
- Frequent snacking – when on a keto diet, this is strongly advised against as that could lead to a spike in insulin levels and it would reduce the effects that help in weight loss.

Identifying the Ketosis Effects

There are several chemical changes, a series of them, happening in your body when the ketosis process occurs.

If left uninitiated, it will become tough to recognize the changes and you may not figure out that ketosis has started in your body. Some of the common characteristics of the effects are the following:

Appetite Suppression

When you only eat vegetables and proteins throughout the keto diet, you will experience your appetite reducing and suppressing itself. This is great for anyone who has issues like frequent snacking, etc.

Loss of Weight

At first, you will experience a lot of weight loss, really fast. This quick dive in your weight is the result of the store of carbohydrates in your body being used up. After this phase of rapid weight loss, it will slow down. It will turn into a slow but sure process, and it is very consistent if you keep following the keto diet properly. Also be sure to keep a check on your calories.

Keto Fever

There is a possibility you will start feeling sick, tired and experience a little brain fog. But fret not – it is a temporary effect. This happens solely because the body starts burning its stores of fat, unlike its previous, regular routine of using carbs as a source of energy. Once you get used to your new routine of no-carbs, your body's level of sugar will stabilize to an extent where it helps eliminate whatever keto fever symptoms you are going through.

Bad Breath

This is probably one of the most eminent symptoms when you enter ketosis. Your breath might adapt an odor that is kind of fruity, as a direct result of the ketone levels increasing. The reason behind that is a kind of ketone, which can be found in your urine and also your breath. This kind of ketone is called acetone.

Even if it may seem like an antagonist to your social life, this effect of bad breath is, in fact, a good symptom that your diet is progressing the right way. To combat this effect, you can chew gum, but make sure you check the listed ingredients.

Chapter Three: How Keto Affects and Benefits Your Body

Manages Blood Sugar Levels

As mentioned earlier, carbohydrates are the reason behind glucose being released into your bloodstream. This is why consuming carbohydrates instantly results in your levels of energy surging up. The hormone insulin regulates your levels of blood sugar. But for some people, insulin functions in a different way. It fails to regulate the levels of blood sugar and that leads to Type II Diabetes. When insulin fails to function the way it is supposed to, it is called insulin resistance.

So, in the case of you being resistant to insulin, the keto diet can greatly help relieve the risk of Type II Diabetes. This is directly a result of the sugar amount releasing into the bloodstream because you reduced your consumption of carbs. So even in the scenario of your insulin failing to do its job, there will be no reason for you to worry over Type II Diabetes.

Even if someone is suffering from Type II Diabetes, they can take up this diet as it will help manage it and you will require a minimal amount of medication.

Blood Pressure Levels Being Regulated

Hypertension has turned into a common issue in the households of many lately. It also increases the risk of a lot disorders and they can be related to cardiac, kidney disorders, and some others. As a result, it is impossible not to acknowledge the seriousness of hypertension.

Reducing one's consumption of salt is one of the most commonly prescribed suggestions by physicians, in order to treat hypertension - all because salt can be instrumental in the increase of your levels of blood pressure.

Wait! Before you feel disheartened at the prospect of removing salt from your diet or having to put up with salt-less food, read on ahead –

With the keto diet, your blood sugar levels will be managed without you having to reduce your salt intake in any manner.

Here's how it works:

- Your levels of blood sugar increase by default, as a result of the consumption of foods that are high in carbohydrates. If you are resistant to insulin and your blood sugar levels are surging up, the outcome is your blood vessels getting constricted. This directly impacts your levels of blood pressure and nudges it to rise up. A reduction in your intake of carbohydrates helps manage your blood sugar levels. There is hardly any reason to worry about hypertension or blood vessels getting constricted when you have brought your blood sugar levels under control.

- Insulin resistance is another crucial reason of hypertension. Soon it will be explained to you how all the visceral fat stocked up in your body can be reduced with the help of the keto diet. Reducing the visceral fat amounts helps manage your resistance towards insulin, which in turn helps lower any factors of risk involved in some cardiac disorders. Managing your insulin resistance means the reduction of one factor of risk in the case of hypertension.
- As you are already aware, your body is encouraged to burn its stores of fat on this diet. When this burning takes place, the potassium and sodium present in your kidneys are cleansed out. This leads to an imbalance of electrolytes, and that can be remedied by increasing your consumption of chicken broth and salt. As must be apparent to you by now, this diet helps manage hypertension without nudging you to reduce your salt intake.

Triglyceride Levels are reduced

An increase in the amount of triglycerides existing in the bloodstream by default ups the risks for many cardiac related disorders. The more you consume carbohydrates, the more the triglyceride levels will go up. As you are aware, carbs convert into glucose and are channeled into your bloodstream as the source of energy.

When there is an excessive amount of glucose in your bloodstream, although the body has already sourced its energy, then the pancreas secretes insulin, which converts the excess but residual glucose into what we call triglycerides.

These then travel to the fat cells. When you aren't consuming foods, the body sources its energy from the store of triglycerides that are released.

Simply put – increased intake of carbohydrates makes way to the levels of triglycerides being increased.

Removal of Visceral Fat

When the foods you have consumed are digested, the fat settles in various parts of your body. This is quite risky because depending on the location of the fat deposits; the factors of risk will tend to vary. Upon consumption the fats are stored in two different places - subcutaneous fat is the fat that is deposited under your skin and visceral fat that is stored on your stomach.

Out of the two, you need to be very careful about visceral fat. It is really dangerous and can negatively affect the quality of the life you are leading. It can also impact the way your organs tend to function. If the amount of visceral fat stored in your body increases, it can lead to organ inflammation, metabolism impairment, and also insulin resistance.

When your metabolism is attacked, it could also affect and negate the efforts you are putting into losing weight. In fact, it could slow down the entire process of weight loss. And that is why it is so important to ensure your deposits of visceral fat are manageable.

The keto diet helps reduce the amount of visceral fat that gets stored up in your body as the diet forces the body to digest this stubborn fat to source energy from. When you get rid of the excess amounts of visceral fat, you automatically reduce the factors of risk for many health disorders. It also stops your weight loss efforts from being rendered useless due to the presence of this fat.

The keto diet is capable of reducing the visceral fat stored in our bodies. This stubborn fat is digested by the body to derive energy. By getting rid of excess visceral fat, you are actually reducing your risk factors of various health disorders. Your efforts to lose weight will also not be compromised by visceral fat's unwanted presence.

Appetite Regulation

This is one of the best aspects of the keto diet – it does not make you feel like you're starving, at least, after the first initial days, once your body starts getting accustomed to sourcing its energy from fat. As a result of this burning of fat to fuel the body, you start feeling more energetic, and the high content of fat in the diet, ensures you are always feeling full.

The keto diet never lets you feel like you are actually on any kind of a diet as it allows you to have all of your favorite foods, with the exception of carbohydrates (and in the case of this book – dairy, as well).

The thing about fats is that it takes time to digest, as opposed to carbohydrates; which is why you end up not feeling hungry too often.

When you are on a carbohydrate specific diet, like any regular diet, your body ends up burning all those carbs really quick and, as a result, you find yourself victimized by frequent hunger pangs.

By following the keto diet, you are eliminating the chances of random and frequent hunger pangs, not to mention the regulation of your appetite also helps in weight loss. Because you are feeling hungry less often, this means eating less than you are used to.

As a result, your only concern becomes reduced burning amounts of calories.

Helps Increase HDL cholesterol level

High Density Lipoprotein is also referred to as good cholesterol. Its job is to ensure that the cholesterol from your food intake goes into the liver. Upon reaching the liver, the cholesterol is either removed from the body or used again by it to derive energy from.

So, HDL cholesterol is instrumental in making sure the content of cholesterol in your food does not clog and create obstructions in our arteries.

As per specific studies, HDL can also be useful in the reduction of inflammation. There are also studies that show the keto diet can largely help improve the HDL levels in your body.

This is due to reducing the consumption of carbohydrates and increasing the intake of healthy fats.

Helps Increase Patterns of LDL cholesterol

LDL cholesterol is commonly referred to and antagonized as the bad cholesterol and can increase the risk of cardiac disorders. There exists a misconception that an increase in LDL cholesterol levels holds the potential to increase your factors of risk for many kinds of cardiac disorders. That, however, is not true. The impact is determined by the size of the particles. As per studies, smaller particles result in greater risks of cardiac disorders.

People who have LDL cholesterol particles that are larger suffer from minimum risk of getting any kind of cardiac disorders. As a result, it is the size of the particles that can decide the factors of risk and their direct relevance to your health and your lifestyle as well.

But this raises the question – how is the keto diet instrumental in enlarging these particles?

Well, every question leads back to the same root of all problems – carbohydrates.

The sizes of these particles are directly linked to the amount of carbohydrates you tend to consume. The vaster the amount of carbs consumed, the smaller the size of these particles will become. When they keep getting smaller, the factors of risk of cardiac disorders will be increasing with each passing day. So, when you opt for a diet like the keto diet, what happens is that you are restricting your intake of carbs in all manners possible, and that also means helping your body deal with all the problems the vast amount of carbs have previously caused or were going to cause.

Thus, when you reduce your intake of carbs, you are nudging the size of these particles to increase and help decrease risk factors of cardiac disorders.

Other Health Benefits

Helps Strengthen Eyes

High levels of sugar can be very toxic and have damaging effects on your eyesight. It also increases your risk of cataracts. But when you follow a diet that has little next to no sugar in it, these risks are instantly eliminated.

Treats Gastrointestinal Issues

Acid reflux, irritable bowel syndrome, heartburn, gallstones and bloating are all problems related to digestion and they can leads to other serious problems if not put under control in time. One of the best methods to handle these issues is by making radical changes in your eating habits and overall diet. A diet that is low-carb directly deals with the origin of these issues. A keto diet helps you improve your eating habits and eases whatever pains you could be experiencing because of enteric problems.

Treats Brain Disorders

Traditionally, long before the keto diet started gaining any popularity for its wide array of benefits, it was actually used as a method to treat epilepsy in children who failed to respond to medication. To function, the brain requires carbohydrates, but thankfully it can also work with ketones, that are generated when the carbohydrates intake is drastically decreased.

Acne

Consuming vast amounts of carbohydrates is deleterious for your skin, and the near absolute absence of carbohydrates in the ketogenic diet automatically helps cleanse your skin. As a result, it improves the overall health of your skin and also makes it glow and evens it out. It is also helpful in reducing skin problems like lesions and inflammation.

Enhanced Mental Focus

As perplexing as it might sound to some, the keto diet can largely help strengthen your mental performance, as ketones are an essential energy source for the brain. They also enhance our focus and our brain's capacity to perform well.

Boosts Women's Health

The keto diet can help in strengthening and improving fertility. Its low-carb factor can also effectively help treat and control the hormonal disorders like PCOS (Polycystic Ovarian Syndrome) that some women face – in fact; the diet can also help in overcoming symptoms such as obesity, acne and irregular menstrual cycles.

Boosts Energy Levels

When carbohydrates turn into glucose and become the main source of energy for our bodies, they make us feel rather tired and fatigued. But fats are a much more feasible power source for the body, and they keep us from feeling lethargic. As they are quite fulfilling, they make sure we are sated and full for lengthy time periods.

Teeth and Gum Protection

When we consume less amounts of sugar, the pH level of the mouth remains normal and that prevents a specific kind of bacteria from breeding. The bacteria is behind gum infections and tooth decay. If you suffer from any kind of gum disease, being 3 months on the keto diet will help decrease it a lot.

Chapter Four: Dairy-free: What, Why, and How

What

People who decide to go for a dairy-free diet or choose to do a diet but without dairy (such dairy-free keto), they do it for their own set of reasons. Some do it to deal with health issues like bloating, digestion problems, skin issues, respiratory conditions and other things that stem from the consumption of dairy products.

As per studies, thirty million to fifty million Americans suffer from lactose intolerance. Thankfully, there exist enough plant based foods and other foodstuffs that are dairy-free to fulfill your body's nutritional needs.

Simply put – a dairy-free diet is a diet that is devoid of milk and any products made from it or have milk as one of their ingredients.

People who are intolerant towards lactose might opt for removing or reducing foods from their diet that contain any amount of lactose.

It might be possible for some to have small portions of food products that contain milk proteins; they might discover their digestive systems finds a fermented form of dairy easier to digest. Those with an allergy related to cow's milk based foods should absolutely remove milk proteins from their food intake and look for alternatives for food allergies that can provide them with calcium and other essential nutrients.

All prime sources of dairy you need to stay away from when going for a dairy-free diet are – milk, butter, cheese, cream, sour cream, cottage cheese, puddings, gelato, whey, casein, custards and sherbet.

Why

If you are wondering why exactly a dairy-free diet is beneficial for you, read on ahead about all the benefits:

Better Digestion

If estimations are anything to go by, of the entire world's population, around 75% has lactose intolerance to some degree. When you follow a diet that is dairy-free and make sure to stick to it, you can successfully avoid digestive symptoms, so many people suffer from on a daily basis.

Removing dairy from your diet can help relieve stomach pain, cramps, gas, bloating, nausea and diarrhea. Dairy has also been observed as key in triggering symptoms of Irritable Bowel Syndrome and other digestive problems.

Clears Your Skin

As per studies, the presence of anabolic steroids and growth hormones in milk add to milk's potential as a stimulant in the case of acne. When you dairy-free and also take some probiotic supplements, it can help in treating acne in a natural manner, without resolving to medications that are harsh on both your skin and health and come with a variety of side-effects.

Reduced Bloating

Dairy products are a common reason behind complaints of bloating among those who are sensitive to dairy or are allergic to it. On its own, bloating is generally an issue with digestion. For a lot of people, the reason behind excessive gas in their intestines, which is how bloating occurs, is because of insufficient digestion of protein – which is an inability of breaking down carbohydrates and sugars completely, and imbalances in gut related bacteria.

These factors are probably due to dairy sensitivities or allergic reactions to them. Following a dairy-free diet can be helpful in getting rid of a bloated tummy.

Reduces Oxidative Stress

It makes sense why diets that are rich in milk and milk-based products are promoted so rigorously. It is mostly to reduce the chances of osteoporotic fractures, which would, in turn, result in the reduction of health care costs.

As per research, consuming high amounts of milk could have unwanted effects, as milk is D-galactose's primary dietary source. D-galactose impacts the process of inflammation and oxidative stress.

According to evidence in several species of animals, a chronic form of exposure to D-galactose is harmful to health. In fact, a low dose of D-galactose triggers changes that are similar to natural aging processes in animals, along with a lifespan that has been shortened as a result of chronic inflammation, oxidative stress damage, decreased immune system, and neurodegeneration.

Reduced Risk of Cancer

As per some research, consumption of milk products can increase one's cancer developing risks. A calcium intake that is high, and mainly sourced from dairy products, can increase the risk of prostate cancer as it lowers a hormone's concentration, a hormone that is believed to protect us against prostate cancer.

There might also be contaminant like pesticides present in milk products, and these have been observed to encourage the cell growth of breast cancer.

A lot of people refuse to believe it, but cancer has a real link to our eating habits. And since it appears to alleviate the risk of some forms of cancer in specific people, opting for a dairy-free diet could help reduce the risks of some types of cancer.

Good for the Respiratory System

Consuming excess amounts of milk has been linked to asthma and increase mucus production in the respiratory tract. People with dairy sensitivities or allergies often report respiratory symptoms – staying away could help people with such problems.

Helps Milk Sensitivity and Allergy

There exists no true cure for being allergic to milk, except for avoiding it entirely along with other milk-based products. Digestive enzymes and probiotics can help people in digesting the proteins in milk a bit better but only in the case of their allergy not being severe. However, for the majority, removing dairy entirely from their diet is the only solution.

For those who are intolerant towards lactose, a lack of or reducing lactase could lead to unabsorbed lactose passing into the colon, which could lead to fermentation of bacteria which in turn would give rise to symptoms such as diarrhea, flatulence, nausea and bloating.

According to a lot of studies, such gastrointestinal symptoms are improved when the diet is entirely cleansed of milk.

Another allergy that is identified as an issue in infancy and could affect about 15% of infants is milk protein allergy. As per speculation, when the mother consumes milk protein, it is passed onto the infant during breastfeeding. Because of this, mothers are often recommended by mom to remove dairy from their diet if their infants show any negative reactions to breast milk.

Now that you have read about both the benefits of the keto diet, and the benefits of going dairy-free, don't you think the combined benefits turn both into a dynamic duo? If you think about all the way your health can attain its best by doing a dairy-free keto diet, wait until you reach the recipes section of this book. They are exactly what you need to get started on your dairy-free keto journey.

How

So far there does not exist any therapies suitable to treat allergies against cow's milk, other than removing it from your diet completely. As a result, being aware of dairy alternative is quite important.

The nutrients that we are at the risk of losing out on by eliminating dairy are calcium, magnesium, and potassium.

Goat Milk

It still is dairy, yes, but it is high in its content of fatty acids and is a lot easier to absorb and assimilate into the body as opposed to cow's milk. Goat milk has a lot concentration of lactose and the particles of fat in this milk are also smaller. As its casein levels are reduced, it becomes a better option for people who are sensitive to casein protein.

It might surprise you, but goat's milk is nutritionally just as high, as it has a high amount of calcium – it can supply thirty-three percent of your everyday value, along with that it is rich in vitamin B2, Vitamin A, potassium, phosphorus, and magnesium.

Coconut Milk

It is globally acclaimed as one of the best options when you go dairy-free. It's natural liquid present in mature coconuts. The milk is in the 'meat' of the coconut, which, when blended, gives us the thick coconut milk. It is 100% devoid of lactose, soy and dairy. Even though cow's milk offers more calcium as opposed to coconut milk, it can be made up for with foods that are rich in calcium, such as broccoli, kale, bok choy, etc.

However, it is worthy to note, coconut milk is high in fat and calories. Although the fat is of a healthier type, it is essential you are mindful of the portion especially if trying to lose weight.

Almond Milk

The nutritional aspects of almonds are many and just as essential. Not only are they rich with their content of unsaturated fatty acids, but also they are low in saturated fatty acids. They have filling fiber, protective and unique Phytosterols antioxidants, and also plant protein.

Almond milk also has probiotic components that can help with detoxification, digestions, and healthy growth of bacteria in the gut flora that is vital in the utilization of nutrients sourced from food and prevents nutritional deficiencies.

Chapter Five: The Dos and Don'ts of Food on Keto

Every diet you will ever come across will have an elaborate list of what you can or cannot eat while on the diet. That is kind of the whole point of a diet.

Anyway, the ketogenic diet is no different. It too has some dos and don'ts. But one of the best aspects is how the section of what's allowed is always greater than what is restricted. If you truly want to benefit from the keto diet and all the amazing impacts it can have on your life, try to stick to these dos and don'ts for the best results.

What to Eat

Meat, fatty fish, eggs:

The keto diet is a diet that is rich in meat content. It allows you to consume a vast variety of meats such as – ham, steak, turn, bacon, chicken, red meat, sausage, etc. Other than that, you are also allowed to consume fish that are high in natural fats. It is advisable to opt for trout, tuna, mackerel, salmon, etc. You can also consume eggs but make sure they are pastured eggs as they are rich in omega-3 and it is a component that can benefit you when you are on the keto diet.

Vegetables that have low carb content:

Opt for vegetables like tomatoes, peppers, onions, lettuce, broccoli, spinach, chives, celery stalk, endive, bamboo shoots, chard, radishes, bok choy, zucchini, cucumber, asparagus, etc. Try to avoid vegetables that are starchy, such as potatoes, sweet potatoes, etc.

Fruits:

Avocado, and for occasional consumption – mulberries, strawberries, blueberries, raspberries, olives, cranberries, and coconut.

Nuts and Seeds:

Pumpkin seeds, flaxseeds, almonds, walnuts, chia seeds, pecans, hazelnuts, sesame seeds, macadamia nuts, etc. are allowed.

(If you are NOT doing a dairy-free keto)

Cream, cheese, and butter:

Grass-fed butter, cheese but the unprocessed varieties – goat cheese, blue cheese, cheddar cheese, cream cheese and mozzarella cheese, etc.

Condiments:

Pepper, herbs, salt, pesto, mayonnaise, lemon or lime zest and juice, and other spices, etc.

Beverages:

Tea – herbal or black, coffee – black or with coconut milk, etc. If you are using dairy, you can add cream to your coffee.

Healthy Oils:

During the keto diet, it is essential to opt for oils that are healthy and help amplify the effects of the diet. You can go for – extra-virgin olive oil, avocado oil and coconut oil, etc.

Chapter Six: Dairy-free Ketogenic Breakfast Recipes

Celery Root Rosti (Hash Browns)

Serves: 3-4

Ingredients:

- 3-4 celery roots, peeled, grated
- Salt to taste
- Pepper to taste
- 2 tablespoons coconut oil

Serving options (optional): Use any

- Tomato salsa
- Scrambled eggs
- Roasted vegetables

Method:

1. Sprinkle salt and pepper over the celery root.
2. Place a pan over medium high heat. Add oil. When the oil melts, add celery root. Spread it all over the pan to make one large one or else make smaller sized hash browns. Smaller sized ones can be cooked in batches.
3. Cook until underside is cooked and golden brown.
4. Flip sides and cook the other side too.
5. Chop into wedges.
6. Serve with any of the suggested options or any other keto friendly, dairy-free options of your choice.

Breakfast Biscuit

Serves: 2

Ingredients:

- 2 tablespoons coconut flour
- A pinch sea salt
- 2 teaspoons coconut oil
- ¼ cup golden flaxseed meal
- 1 teaspoon aluminum-free baking powder
- 2 large eggs, beaten

Method:

1. Add all the dry ingredients into a bowl.
2. Add coconut oil and mix well until crumbly in texture. Add egg and mix well.
3. Grease 2 small ovenproof bowls or ramekins and add the mixture into the bowls.
4. Bake in a preheated oven at 350° F for about 15 minutes or until firm.
5. Alternately, you can microwave it on high for about 55 seconds.
6. When done, cool on a cooling rack.
7. Serve.

Spinach Omelet with Egg whites

Serves: 2

Ingredients:

- 2 yolks
- 10 egg whites
- 1 tomato, chopped
- 1 medium onion, chopped
- 1 cup spinach, shredded
- A handful basil, chopped
- 2 cloves garlic, minced
- ¼ cup almond milk
- Cooking spray

Method:

1. Whisk together yolks, whites, along with almond milk in a bowl.
2. Take a nonstick pan and place it over medium heat. Spray with cooking spray. When oil is heated, add onion, tomato and spinach and sauté for a couple of minutes.
3. Remove the vegetables and place on a plate.
4. Spray the pan again with cooking spray. Let the pan heat.
5. Lower heat and pour half the egg mixture into the pan. When the eggs are set, place half the

vegetable mixture on one half of the omelet. Fold the other half over the filling.

6. Remove on to a serving plate and serve.
7. Repeat the above 2 steps with the remaining egg mixture and vegetables to make the other omelet.

Classic Bacon and Eggs

Serves: 2

Ingredients:

- 4 eggs
- 2 ¾ ounces bacon slices
- A handful fresh parsley, chopped
- 4 cherry tomatoes, halved
- Salt to taste
- Pepper to taste

Method:

1. Place a skillet over medium heat. Add bacon and cook until crisp.
2. Remove the bacon from the skillet on some paper towels. When cool enough to handle, chop or break into smaller pieces.
3. Cook eggs with the fat in the skillet, as per your preference.
4. Place eggs and bacon on serving plates. Sprinkle salt and pepper on top and serve.

Coconut Porridge

Serves: 2

Ingredients:

- 2 ounces coconut oil
- 2 tablespoons coconut flour
- 8 tablespoons coconut cream
- 2 eggs
- ½ teaspoon ground psyllium husk powder
- A pinch salt

Method:

1. Add all the ingredients into a nonstick pan and stir.
2. Place the pan over low heat, stirring all the time until you get the desired texture.
3. Garnish with frozen berries and coconut milk or cream if desired and serve.

Fat Bomb Smoothie

Serves: 2

Ingredients:

- 2 cups coconut milk
- 2 tablespoon peanut butter
- 1 teaspoon ground cinnamon
- 4 tablespoons coconut oil
- 1 teaspoon vanilla extract
- Ice cubes, as required

Method:

1. Add coconut milk, peanut butter, cinnamon, coconut oil, vanilla and ice into a blender and blend until smooth.
2. Pour into glasses and serve.
3. For a change in taste, you can add keto friendly non-dairy chocolate protein powder or add a few slices avocado while blending.

Blueberry Smoothie

Serves: 1

Ingredients:

- 1 cup coconut milk
- ½ tablespoon lemon juice
- ¼ cup blueberries, fresh or frozen
- ¼ teaspoon vanilla extract

Method:

1. Add all the ingredients into a blender and blend until smooth.
2. Pour into a tall glass and serve with crushed ice.

Chapter Seven: Dairy-free Ketogenic Snack Recipes

Salty Chocolate Treat

Serves: 5

Ingredients:

- 1 ¾ ounces dairy-free dark chocolate
- 1 tablespoon coconut chips, unsweetened, roasted
- A large pinch flaky salt or to taste
- 5 hazelnuts or pecans or walnuts
- ½ tablespoon pumpkin seeds

Method:

1. Set a double boiler. Add chocolate into a heatproof bowl and place on the double boiler. Stir frequently until chocolate melts.
2. Pour melted chocolate into 5 cupcake liners.
3. Sprinkle nuts, chocolate chips and seeds into the liners.
4. Sprinkle salt op top.
5. Cool completely and refrigerate until use.

Seed Crackers

Serves: 15

Ingredients:

- ¼ cup almond flour
- ¾ teaspoon sea salt
- ¼ cup sesame seeds
- ¼ cup sunflower seeds
- ¼ cup flaxseeds or chia seeds
- ¼ teaspoon pumpkin seeds
- ½ tablespoon psyllium husk powder
- 2 tablespoons coconut oil, melted
- ½ cup boiling water

Method:

1. Mix together almond flour, salt, all the seeds and psyllium husk powder into a bowl. Pour water into the bowl. Form into dough.
2. Line a baking sheet with parchment paper.
3. Place the dough at the center of the paper. Cover with another paper and roll the dough until it is about ½ inch thick.
4. After rolling, cut the dough with a knife into squares.
5. Place the baking sheet in a preheated oven at 350 ^{0} F for about 10-15 minutes until golden brown. Cool and separate the squares.

6. Store in an airtight container.

Zucchini Chips with Smoked Paprika

Serves: 4

Ingredients:

- 2 medium zucchinis
- 1 teaspoon salt or to taste
- 4 tablespoons olive oil
- 2 teaspoons smoked paprika
- ½ teaspoon pepper powder to taste

Method:

1. Cut the zucchini into ¼ inch thick slices, crosswise with a mandolin slicer or a knife.
2. Place the zucchini in a colander in layers sprinkled with salt and pepper. Set aside for an hour.
3. Pat dry the zucchini slices with a paper towel and place on a baking tray that is lined with parchment paper. Brush the parchment paper with oil.
4. Brush the top of the slices with oil. Sprinkle paprika and pepper.
5. Bake in a preheated oven at 250° F for 45 minutes. Turn off the oven and let the chips remain inside for an hour.
6. Cool completely.
7. Transfer into airtight container.

Zesty Nacho Kale Chips

Serves: 4-6

Ingredients:

- 4 large bunch kale, discard stems and hard ribs, torn into bite size pieces
- 1 cup tahini
- ½ cup nutritional yeast
- 1 large red bell pepper, chopped
- 2 tablespoons golden balsamic vinegar (optional)
- 2 teaspoons garlic powder
- 1 teaspoon pepper powder or to taste
- 1 cup sunflower seed butter
- 1 cup apple cider vinegar
- ½ cup lemon juice or to taste
- 4 tablespoons sesame oil or olive oil
- 2-3 drops stevia (optional)
- 1 tablespoon coconut aminos or tamari
- 1 teaspoon onion powder
- 1 teaspoon salt or to taste
- Cooking spray

Method:

1. Sprinkle salt on the kale. Spray with cooking spray. Keep it aside for a while.
2. Spread the leaves on a greased baking sheet.

3. Bake in a preheated oven at 250° F until crisp. It may take a couple of hours.
4. Meanwhile, add rest of the ingredients into a blender and blend until smooth.
5. Pour sauce into a large bowl.
6. When the chips are ready, add chips into the bowl of sauce. Toss with tongs and serve right away.
7. If you are not using all the chips and sauce, store in separate airtight containers. Refrigerate the sauce until use. Remove from the refrigerator 40-50 minutes before serving. Add kale chips, toss and serve.

Broccoli Tots

Makes: 40-50

Ingredients:

- 4 medium heads broccoli, cut into florets
- 1 cup yellow bell pepper, finely chopped
- 1 cup almond meal
- Salt to taste
- Freshly ground pepper to taste
- 1 cup onion, finely chopped
- 2 egg whites
- 2 eggs
- A handful fresh parsley, chopped
- Cooking spray

Method:

1. Spray a baking sheet with cooking spray.
2. Place a large pot, half filled with water over medium high heat.
3. When the water begins to boil, add salt and broccoli. Cook for 4-5 minutes or until tender.
4. Drain and transfer into the food processor bowl. Pulse until very fine.
5. Squeeze out as much as moisture as possible from the broccoli and add into a bowl.
6. Add rest of the ingredients and mix well.

7. Shape into tots using about 1-2 tablespoons of the mixture.
8. Place on the prepared baking sheet.
9. Bake in a preheated oven at 375° F until crisp.
10. Serve with a keto friendly dip of your choice.

Avocado Hummus

Serves: 5-6

Ingredients:

- 2 ripe avocados, peeled, pitted, roughly chopped
- A large handful fresh cilantro, chopped
- 2 tablespoons lemon juice
- 3 tablespoons sunflower seeds
- 3 tablespoons olive oil
- 5 teaspoons tahini paste
- ½ teaspoon ground cumin
- 1 small clove garlic, peeled,
- Salt to taste
- Pepper to taste
- Water, if required

Method:

1. Add all the ingredients into a blender and blend until smooth. Add water if the hummus is very thick. Blend again.
2. Transfer into a bowl. Taste and adjust the seasoning and oil if required.
3. Serve.
4. Serving options: With keto friendly crackers, cucumber sticks, in wraps, as a side dish, etc.

Chapter Eight: Dairy-free Keto Side Dish Recipes

Rutabaga Curls

Serves: 2

Ingredients:

- ¾ pound rutabaga
- ½ tablespoon paprika or chili powder
- 6-7 teaspoons olive oil
- ½ teaspoon salt

Method:

1. Make noodles of the rutabaga using a spiralizer. You can also make noodles using a julienne peeler or with a sharp knife. Cut into bite size pieces.
2. Add the noodles into a bowl. Add rest of the ingredients and toss well.
3. Transfer on to a baking sheet. Spread it evenly.
4. Bake in a preheated oven at 450° F for about 10 minutes.
5. Serve right away.

Coleslaw

Serves: 8

Ingredients:

- 1 medium green cabbage, thinly sliced
- 2 teaspoons salt
- ¼ teaspoon fennel seeds (optional)
- 2 tablespoons Dijon mustard
- Juice of a lemon
- ¾ cup mayonnaise or to taste
- Pepper to taste

Method:

1. Add cabbage into a colander. Add salt and lemon juice and mix well.
2. Let it sit in the colander for 10 minutes.
3. Add cabbage back into the bowl. Add rest of the ingredients. Mix well.
4. Serve.

Roasted Radishes with Rosemary

Serves: 4

Ingredients:

- 6 cups radishes, quartered if large in size else halved, chop the leaves and keep aside
- 1 teaspoons sea salt or to taste
- 15 whole black peppercorns
- 6 sprigs fresh rosemary, chopped
- 6 tablespoon olive oil

Method:

1. Add salt and peppercorns into a mortar and pestle and crush the peppercorns.
2. Place together in a bowl, radishes, 4 tablespoons oil, rosemary and the crushed pepper. Toss well.
3. Transfer on to a greased baking sheet. Spread it in a single layer.
4. Roast in a preheated oven at 425° F until crisp and brown.
5. Meanwhile, place a skillet over medium heat. Add the remaining oil. When the oil is heated, add the radish leaves, a little salt and sauté until the leaves are wilted.
6. Add the roasted radish and stir well.
7. Serve right away.

Roasted Fennel with Lemon and Sugar snaps

Serves: 2

Ingredients:

- Juice of ½ lemon
- 1 ½ tablespoons olive oil
- 1 tablespoon sunflower seeds or pumpkin seeds, roasted
- ½ pound fresh fennel, chopped into wedges
- 2 ¾ ounces sugar snaps, shredded
- Pepper to taste
- Salt to taste

Method:

1. Place fennel in a baking dish. Pour oil over it. Toss well. Sprinkle salt and pepper and toss well.
2. Squeeze the juice from the lemon and use in some other recipe. Cut the lemon rind into 3-4 pieces and place it in the baking dish, all around the fennel pieces.
3. Roast in a preheated oven at 450° F for 20-30 minutes or until golden brown in color.
4. Add sugar snap peas and pumpkin seeds and mix well.
5. Goes well as a side with chicken, fish, lamb, pork, turkey or beef.

Fried Green Cabbage

Serves: 2

Ingredients:

- ¾ pound green cabbage, shredded
- Salt to taste
- Pepper to taste
- 1 ½ ounces coconut oil

Method:

1. Place a skillet over medium heat. Add oil. When oil melts, add cabbage and sauté until the cabbage is cooked as per your desire. Lower heat halfway through cooking. Stir frequently.
2. Add salt and pepper and mix well.
3. Serve hot.

Celery Root and Cauliflower Puree with Garlicky Greens

Serves: 2-3

Ingredients:

For celery root and cauliflower puree:

- 1 celery root of about 8 ounces, peeled, cut into cubes of ½ inch each
- ¼ teaspoon salt
- 8 ounces cauliflower, cut into small florets
- 1 ½ tablespoons extra -virgin olive oil

For sautéed chard:

- 1 bunch Swiss chard, rinsed, cut leaves into strips and thinly cut the stems up to ¾ the stems
- 1 small clove garlic, minced
- Sea salt to taste
- ½ tablespoon extra-virgin olive oil
- A pinch red pepper flakes

Method:

1. To make celery root and cauliflower puree: Steam the celery roots and cauliflower in the steaming equipment you have. Steam until tender.
2. Place the steamed vegetables into a food processor. Add a couple of tablespoons of the

cooked liquid, salt and oil. Blend until the texture you desire is achieved.

3. Cover and keep warm.
4. To make sautéed chard: Place a skillet over medium heat. Add oil. When the oil is heated, add garlic and red pepper flakes and sauté for a few seconds until fragrant.
5. Add chard leaves and stems and sauté for 2-3 minutes.
6. Cover and cook for some more time until tender. Add salt and stir.
7. Serve celery root and cauliflower puree over the sautéed chard.

Cauliflower Rice

Serves: 2-3

Ingredients:

- ¾ pound cauliflower, chopped into florets
- 1 onion, finely diced (optional)
- 4 tablespoons olive oil or coconut oil
- 4 cloves garlic, minced (optional)
- ¼ teaspoon turmeric powder (optional)
- Salt to taste
- Pepper powder to taste

Method:

1. Add the cauliflower florets into the food processor and pulse until you get a rice like texture. You can also grate the cauliflower.
2. Place a large nonstick skillet over medium high heat. Add oil. When the oil is heated, add onions and sauté until translucent. Add garlic and sauté until fragrant. Add turmeric powder and sauté for 5-8 seconds.
3. Add cauliflower rice and sauté for about 5-6 minutes. Remove from heat.
4. Sprinkle salt and pepper just before serving.
5. If you are not using the optional ingredients, you can also cook in the microwave by adding cauliflower rice into a microwave safe bowl.

Cover the bowl with plastic wrap. Microwave on high for 5-6 minutes.

6. Unwrap and add oil and salt. Mix well and serve.

Roasted Tomato Salad

Serves: 2-3

Ingredients:

- ¾ pound cherry tomatoes
- ½ teaspoon sea salt
- 1 scallion, sliced
- 1 ½ tablespoons olive oil
- ¼ teaspoon pepper
- ½ tablespoon red wine vinegar

Method:

1. Pour oil on the cherry tomatoes and toss well. Add salt and pepper and toss well.
2. Grill or roast in an oven until the tomatoes begin to get soft and charred.
3. Transfer on to a plate. Place scallions on top. Drizzle vinegar and some more oil if desired and serve.

Celeriac "Grits"

Serves: 4

Ingredients:

- 4 medium celeriac's, trim the outer brown layer, cubed
- 2 tablespoons pure avocado oil
- 1 teaspoon pepper powder
- 4 cups chicken stock
- 2 medium onion, chopped
- 2 teaspoons sea salt or to taste
- 4 cloves garlic, minced

Method:

1. Add the celeriac to the food processor and pulse until you get corn grit like texture. You can also grate the cauliflower.
2. Place a large nonstick skillet over medium high heat. Add oil. When the oil is heated, add onions and sauté until translucent. Add garlic and sauté until fragrant.
3. Add rest of the ingredients into the skillet and stir.
4. Cover and cook for 10-12 minutes. Uncover and cook until most of the liquid is absorbed.
5. Serve hot.

Chapter Nine: Dairy-free Ketogenic Main Course Recipes

Cream of Chicken Soup

Serves: 4

Ingredients:

- 2 medium cauliflowers, broken into florets
- 2 cups chicken broth
- 1 teaspoon sea salt
- Freshly ground pepper to taste
- ¼ teaspoon dried thyme
- ½ cup chicken thighs, cooked, finely chopped
- 1 1/3 cups almond milk, unsweetened
- 2 teaspoons onion powder
- ½ teaspoon garlic powder
- ¼ teaspoon celery seeds (optional)
- ½ cup Collagen protein beef gelatin (optional)

Method:

1. Set aside the chicken and gelatin and add rest of the ingredients into a soup pot.

2. Place the soup pot over medium heat. Cover with a lid and let it boil.
3. Lower heat when it begins to boil. Simmer until cauliflower is soft.
4. Turn off the heat. Take out about a cup of the cooked liquid and add into a bowl.
5. Add a teaspoon of gelatin at a time into the bowl of cooked liquid. Whisk well each time until the gelatin is dissolved. Continue doing this until the entire gelatin is added.
6. Pour the gelatin mixture into a blender. Also, add the cooked cauliflower mixture.
7. Blend until smooth and creamy.
8. Pour the soup back into the pot. Place the pot over low heat.
9. Add chicken and stir. Cover and cook until the soup is heated thoroughly.
10. Ladle into soup bowls and serve.

Cabbage Soup with Chicken Quenelles

Serves: 8

Ingredients:

- 2 pounds ground chicken
- 2 tablespoons dried parsley
- 1 teaspoon salt
- 2 chicken cubes
- 2 pounds green cabbage or savoy cabbage
- Salt to taste
- Pepper to taste
- 2 eggs
- 2 teaspoons onion powder
- ½ teaspoon ground nutmeg
- 8 cups water
- 4 ounces coconut oil
- 2 chicken bouillon cubes

For parsley butter:

- 10 ounces coconut oil, at room temperature
- Salt to taste
- Pepper to taste
- 2 tablespoons fresh parsley, minced

Method:

1. Add parsley, coconut oil, salt and pepper into a bowl. Mix well.

2. To make quenelles: Add chicken, salt, pepper, garlic powder, onion powder and eggs into a bowl and mix well.
3. Chill for 15-20 minutes in the refrigerator.
4. Make small balls of the mixture of about 2.5 cm diameter.
5. Place a soup pot over medium high heat. Add coconut oil. When the coconut oil melts, add cabbage and sauté until light golden brown.
6. Add chicken bouillon cubes and water and stir. When it begins to boil, lower heat.
7. Drop the quenelles, one at a time into the simmering broth. Let it simmer for 10-15 minutes or until the quenelle are cooked.
8. Ladle into soup bowls. Top with a blob of parsley butter and serve.

Thai Chicken Skillet

Serves: 6

Ingredients:

- 3 tablespoons coconut oil
- 1 ½ cups chicken stock
- 6 large bone-in chicken thighs trimmed of excess fat and skin
- ½ cup onion, chopped
- 3 cloves garlic, minced
- 9 ounces green bell pepper, chopped
- 3 tablespoons lime juice
- 1 ½ cups coconut milk
- Salt to taste
- Pepper to taste
- 2 tablespoons Thai curry paste or more to taste
- Cauliflower rice to serve

Toppings: Optional

- Handful fresh cilantro, chopped
- Lime juice
- Red chili pepper, sliced

Method:

1. Place a large skillet over high heat. Add 1-½ tablespoons of oil. When oil melts, place chicken with its skin side down, in a single layer.
2. Lower heat to medium high heat and cook for 5 minutes. Flip sides and cook for 3 minutes.

3. Remove chicken with a slotted spoon and place on a plate.
4. Add remaining oil into the skillet. Add onion and garlic and sauté until translucent.
5. Add bell pepper and sauté for a minute. Add remaining ingredients and mix well.
6. Add the chicken back into the skillet with the skin side up. Cook for 10-12 minutes.
7. Transfer into a preheated oven. Broil for a few minutes until crisp. Top with optional toppings if desired.
8. Serve with cauliflower rice on the side.

Low Carb Chicken and Vegetable Curry

Serves: 8

Ingredients:

- 2 pounds chicken thighs, boneless, chopped into bite sized pieces if desired
- 2 yellow onions, chopped
- 16 ounces broccoli, cut into smaller florets
- 2 red chili peppers, deseeded, chopped
- 7 ounces fresh green beans, chopped
- 6 tablespoons coconut oil
- 3 ½ cans (14.5 ounces each) coconut milk or coconut cream
- 2 tablespoons red curry paste or to taste
- 2 tablespoons fresh ginger, grated
- ½ teaspoon cayenne pepper or to taste (optional)
- Salt to taste
- Cauliflower rice to serve

Method:

1. Add oil into a Dutch oven or a large saucepan.
2. Add onion, ginger and chili pepper and sauté until onions turn translucent.
3. Stir in the curry paste and chicken. Mix well.
4. Cook until light brown. Add more oil if required.
5. Add vegetables and the thick part of coconut cream and milk. Use the liquid in some other recipe. Cook until done.
6. Serve hot over cauliflower rice.

Italian Meatza

Serves: 8

For the crust:

- 2 pounds lean ground beef
- 2 tablespoons fresh basil chopped or 2 teaspoons dried basil
- 4 tablespoons mixed dried Italian herbs like oregano, thyme, parsley, etc.
- 1 teaspoon salt
- 1 teaspoon black pepper
- 2 cloves garlic, minced
- Fresh basil, chopped to garnish

For topping: Use any, as required (optional)

- 1 cup tomato sauce
- ½ cup sundried tomatoes, sliced
- 1 red bell pepper, sliced
- 10 olives, sliced
- 1 artichoke hearts (canned or packed in oil), chopped
- 1 cup arugula leaves

Method:

1. To make meat crust: Mix together all the ingredients of crust in a bowl.

2. Add the mixture to a large pie pan or into 2 smaller pie pans. Press it well on to the bottom of the pan.
3. Bake in a preheated oven at 400° F for about 15-18 minutes. Drain off the fat that is remaining in the pan.
4. For topping: Spread tomato sauce over the baked beef crusts.
5. Sprinkle toppings and bake for about 8-10 minutes.
6. Cut into wedges and serve.

Steak and Broccoli Stir Fry

Serves: 4

Ingredients:

- 8 ounces coconut oil
- 18 ounces broccoli, chop the florets as well as the stems
- 2 tablespoons tamari sauce (optional)
- Salt to taste
- Pepper to taste
- 1 ½ pounds rib eye steaks, sliced
- 2 yellow onion, sliced
- 2 tablespoons pumpkin seeds

Method:

1. Place a wok or frying pan over medium heat. Add half the oil. When it melts, add steak slices and cook until brown. Sprinkle salt and pepper. Mix well.
2. Remove steaks with a slotted spoon and place on a plate.
3. Add broccoli and onions into the pan. Sauté until broccoli is crisp as well as tender. Add more coconut oil if needed.
4. Add tamari and mix well. Add steak back into the pan and mix well. Taste and adjust the seasonings if necessary.
5. Serve right away with pumpkin seeds.

Pork and Green Pepper Stir Fry

Serves: 4

Ingredients:

- 1 1/3 pound pork shoulder slices
- 4 scallions, sliced
- 4 tablespoons almonds
- Salt to taste
- Pepper to taste
- 4 green bell peppers, sliced
- 8 ounces coconut oil or lard
- 2 teaspoons chili paste

Method:

1. Place a wok or frying pan over medium heat. Add most of the oil.
2. When it melts, add pork and raise the heat to high heat. Cook until brown.
3. Add scallions and bell peppers. Stir and add chili paste. Mix well. Sauté until slightly tender.
4. Add salt and pepper and mix well.
5. Top with almonds and remaining oil and serve right away.

Spicy Pulled Pork

Serves: 3

Ingredients:

- 1 pound pork shoulder
- ½ tablespoon cocoa nibs or cocoa powder
- ¼ teaspoon ground ginger
- ¼ teaspoon anise seeds or fennel seeds
- ¼ tablespoon black pepper powder
- ¼ teaspoon cayenne pepper
- ½ tablespoon salt
- 1 tablespoon olive oil

Method:

1. Add all the spices and cocoa nibs into a grinder and process until fine. You can also pound using a mortar and pestle.
2. Rub this mixture all over the pork. Place in a baking dish or rimmed baking sheet.
3. Bake in a preheated oven at 400° F for a few hours until tender.
4. Alternately, you can cook in a slow cooker.
5. When the pork is done, remove the pork and set aside on your cutting board.
6. When cool enough to handle, shred with a pair of forks.

7. Serve with roasted tomato salad and avocado hummus.

Ground Pork Tacos

Serves: 6 (5 wraps per serving)

Ingredients:

- 2 pounds ground pork
- 1 ½ teaspoons onion powder
- 1 teaspoon ground cumin
- 20 large lettuce leaves or more if required
- 1 ½ teaspoons garlic powder
- 1 teaspoon sea salt
- ½ teaspoon ground pepper or to taste

For toppings:

- ¼ cup salsa
- 2 medium onions, chopped
- ¾ cup green bell pepper, chopped
- ¾ cup red bell pepper, chopped
- Or any other dairy-free keto toppings of your choice

Method:

1. Add pork, garlic powder, onion powder, salt, cumin, and pepper into a bowl. Mix well using your hands.
2. Place the skillet over medium heat. Add the meat mixture. Stir constantly and cook until brown.

3. Remove the pork with a slotted spoon and place in a bowl. Discard the fat that is remaining in the skillet.
4. Add salsa and mix well. Taste and adjust the seasonings if necessary.
5. Lay the lettuce leaves on your working area. Place some pork filling at the center.
6. Sprinkle peppers, and onions. Wrap and serve.

Creamy Cauliflower and Ground Beef Skillet

Serves: 2

Ingredients:

- 1 tablespoon coconut oil
- 1 clove garlic, chopped
- ½ pound lean ground beef
- Freshly cracked pepper to taste
- ¼ cup keto friendly mayonnaise + 2 tablespoons extra to top
- 2 tablespoons toasted sunflower seed butter
- ½ teaspoon fish sauce
- 2 large eggs
- ¼ ripe avocado, peeled, diced
- ½ tablespoon apple cider vinegar
- 2 tablespoons chopped onions
- 2 jalapeños peppers, sliced, divided
- ½ teaspoon Himalayan salt
- ½ pound grated cauliflower
- ¼ cup water
- ½ tablespoon coconut aminos
- ½ teaspoon ground cumin
- A handful fresh parsley, chopped

Method:

1. Place a cast iron skillet or a heavy bottomed skillet over medium high heat.

2. Add coconut oil. When the oil melts, add onion, garlic and half the jalapeño pepper and sauté for a few minutes until slightly soft.
3. Stir in beef, pepper and salt and cook until brown.
4. Reduce heat to medium low and add cauliflower and sauté for a couple of minutes.
5. Add mayonnaise, sun butter, water, coconut aminos, and cumin and fish sauce into a small bowl and whisk well. Pour into the skillet and mix well. Sauté for a few minutes until the mixture is slightly dry.
6. Turn off the heat. Make 2 cavities (big enough for an egg to fit in) in the mixture. Crack an egg into each of the cavity. Season with salt and pepper. Sprinkle the remaining jalapeños pepper slices over it.
7. Transfer the skillet into a preheated oven. Broil for 8-10 minutes until the eggs are cooked as per your liking.
8. Meanwhile, mix together in a bowl, 2 tablespoons mayonnaise and apple cider vinegar. Drizzle over the skillet.
9. Top with avocado and parsley. Pierce the egg yolks and serve.

Pan Grilled Lamb Chops and Cardoons

Serves: 4

Ingredients:

<u>For lamb chops:</u>

- 4 lamb shoulder chops
- 2 sprigs fresh rosemary
- Sea salt to taste
- 6 tablespoons olive oil
- 4 cloves garlic

<u>For cardoons:</u>

- Pepper powder to taste
- Sea salt to taste
- 2 bunches cardoons
-

Method:

1. To make lamb chops: Add garlic, rosemary, oil and salt into a small blender and blend until smooth. Alternately, you can pound in a mortar and pestle.
2. Transfer the mixture into a bowl.
3. Rub the mixture all over the lamb chops and place it in a bowl. Cover and set aside for at least 30 -60 minutes.

4. Place a cast iron skillet over medium heat. Place lamb chops on it. Cook in batches if your skillet is not large enough.
5. Cook for about 5 minutes or until brown. Flip sides and cook the other side too. The internal temperature with a cooking thermometer should register 125° F when the meat is cooked.
6. Remove from the pan and keep warm. Let the juices remain in the skillet.
7. To make cardoons: Rinse the cardoon stems. Using a sharp knife, peel off the outer most layer of the cardoon. Chop into 4 inch pieces.
8. Place a pot of water over medium heat. Add salt and cardoons. Cook until cardoons are tender. Drain.
9. Place the skillet back over heat. Add cardoons to it. Cook cardoons in the juice for a few minutes.
10. Serve cardoons with lamb chops.

Lamb Chops with Lemony Gremolata

Serves: 4

Ingredients:

For Gremolata:

- Zest of 1 lemon, grated
- ½ cup parsley leaves, loosely packed, minced
- 1 clove garlic, minced or pressed

For lamb chops:

- 1 tablespoon olive oil
- 1 tablespoon Gremolata
- ½ rack of lamb, cut into 4 individual rib chops
- Juice of ½ lemon
- Salt to taste
- Pepper to taste
- 1 tablespoon avocado oil

Method:

1. To make Gremolata: Mix together parsley, lemon zest and garlic on your cutting board. Mince the entire ingredients together a few times. Use 1 tablespoon of the Gremolata to make the lamb chops.
2. Add olive oil, 1 tablespoon Gremolata, lemon juice, salt and pepper into a bowl and mix well. Cover and chill for 1-4 hours. Stir a couple of times while it is marinating.

3. Remove from the refrigerator for 30-40 minutes before cooking.
4. Place a skillet over medium heat. Add oil. When the oil is heated, add chops and cook for about 3 minutes on each side for medium rare.
5. Sprinkle remaining Gremolata on top and serve.

Herb-Crusted Lamb Chops Recipe

Serves: 4

Ingredients:

- 4 large cloves garlic, smashed
- 2 sprigs fresh rosemary, snipped
- 2 tablespoons extra-virgin olive oil
- 2 sprigs fresh thyme, snipped
- 8 lamb loin chops (4 ½ inches)

Method:

1. Add garlic, herbs and half the oil into a bowl. Mix well. Add lamb chops and dredge the chops in the mixture.
2. Chill for 30-45 minutes.
3. Place an ovenproof skillet over high heat. Add remaining oil. When the oil is heated, add lamb chops and cook until brown on both the sides. It should take around 3 minutes on each side. Turn off the heat and transfer into a preheated oven
4. Bake at 400° F for about 10 minutes for medium rare.
5. When done, let it sit for 5 minutes.
6. Serve.

Thai Fish with Curry and Coconut

Serves: 2

Ingredients:

- ¾ pound fish fillets, cut crosswise into 1 inch slices
- ½ pound broccoli, cut into florets
- 1-2 tablespoons Thai red or green curry paste
- 7 ounces thick coconut milk or coconut cream
- 2 tablespoons coconut oil
- Sea salt to taste
- Pepper powder to taste
- ¼ cup fresh cilantro, chopped
- Cooking spray

Method:

1. Place fish in a baking dish. Place blobs of coconut oil over the fish at different places.
2. Add coconut milk, cilantro and red curry paste into a bowl and whisk well. Pepper. Pour over the fish.
3. Bake in a preheated oven at 400° F for about 20 minutes or until tender.
4. Meanwhile, steam the broccoli in salted water. Drain and set aside.
5. Serve fish curry with steamed broccoli.

Lemon Garlic Shrimp

Serves: 4

Ingredients:

- 20 large shrimp, peeled, deveined
- Juice of 2 lemons
- 6 cloves garlic, minced
- 1 teaspoon + 2 tablespoons sea salt
- A handful fresh parsley + extra to garnish
- 4 tablespoons 100% pure avocado oil
- 1 teaspoon smoked paprika
- ½ teaspoon + ½ teaspoon pepper powder
- Lemon wedges to serve

Method:

1. Add lemon juice, garlic, avocado oil, paprika, 1 teaspoon salt, paprika, parsley and ½ teaspoon pepper into a bowl. Mix well. Cover and set aside for a while for the flavors to set in.
2. Place a large pot of water with remaining salt over medium heat. Add remaining pepper and stir. Bring to the boil.
3. Add shrimp and simmer until shrimp turns pink. Turn off heat.
4. Drain and add shrimp into the lemon – oil mixture. Cover with foil and set aside for 10 minutes.

5. Serve shrimp over celeriac grits. Garnish with parsley and drizzle some lemon juice on top and serve.

Fish with Vegetables Baked in Foil

Serves: 8

Ingredients:

- 4 pounds white fish fillets, cut into bite size pieces
- 2 yellow onions, chopped
- 4 red bell peppers, sliced
- 2 fresh fennel or pointed cabbage or savoy cabbage, sliced
- 1 cup olives, pitted
- 2 limes, sliced
- 1 cup white wine
- 11 ounces coconut oil
- 1 leek, sliced
- 4 cloves garlic, sliced
- 24 cherry tomatoes, halved
- 2 carrots, peeled, sliced
- 1 cup fresh thyme or fresh parsley, chopped
- Salt to taste
- Pepper to taste
- 6 tablespoons olive oil

For quick aioli:

- 2 cups keto friendly, dairy-free mayonnaise
- Salt to taste
- Pepper to taste
- 2 cloves garlic, minced

Method:

1. Place a large sheet of parchment paper or foil in a roasting pan in such a way that it is hanging out from the pan. You should be able to make a packet in the end.
2. Place the fish in the roasting pan. Spread all the vegetables over the fish, evenly. Sprinkle garlic, salt, lime slices, olives, tomatoes and parsley.
3. Pour oil and dry white wine over it. Dot with coconut oil at different spots on the vegetables.
4. Fold the hanging foil over the filling. Seal it well and tightly. Take another sheet of foil and cover the packet once more.
5. Bake in a preheated oven at 400° F for about 40 minutes.
6. Meanwhile, make the aioli as follows: Add mayonnaise, garlic, salt and pepper into a bowl and mix well.
7. Serve fish and vegetables with a large blob of aioli.
8. Serve right away.

Vegan Pumpkin Risotto

Serves: 6

Ingredients:

- ½ cup leeks, chopped
- 6 cups cauliflower, grated to rice like texture
- ½ cup nutritional yeast
- 4 tablespoons vegan butter or olive oil
- Pepper to taste
- Salt to taste
- 1 cup pureed pumpkin or butternut squash
- 2 teaspoons paprika or to taste
- ½ cup fresh parsley, chopped (option)
- ½ cup vegetable broth or non-dairy milk of your choice

Method:

1. Place a skillet over medium heat. Add vegan butter and melt. Add leeks and sauté until translucent. Add paprika, salt and pepper and stir for a few seconds.
2. Add broth and stir. Add cauliflower and mix well.
3. Cook until the cauliflower turns soft. Stir a couple of times while it is cooking.
4. Add pumpkin puree and mix well. Taste and adjust the seasoning if necessary.
5. Add nutritional yeast and stir.
6. Garnish with parsley and stir.

Vegan Coconut Lime Noodles with Chili Tamari Tofu

Serves: 2

Ingredients:

For noodles:

- 7 ounces canned full fat coconut milk
- 2 tablespoons sesame seeds
- ¼ teaspoon ground or fresh ginger, grated
- Salt to taste
- 1 package (8 ounces) shirataki noodles
- Juice of ½ lime
- Zest of ½ lime, grated + extra to garnish
- A large pinch red pepper flakes, to garnish

For tofu:

- 7 ounces extra firm tofu, drained, pressed of excess moisture, cut into 1" cubes
- ½ tablespoon olive oil
- 2 tablespoons low sodium tamari
- Cayenne pepper to taste

Method:

1. Place tofu in a shallow dish in a single layer. Mix together in a bowl, oil, tamari and cayenne pepper and pour over the tofu. Toss well so that it is well coated.

2. Transfer on to a baking sheet. Spread it in a single layer.
3. Bake in a preheated oven at 350° F for about 20-25 minutes.
4. Meanwhile, drain the noodles. Rinse and add into a wok or skillet.
5. Place the skillet over medium heat. Add rest of the ingredients of the noodles and mix well. Cover the pan partially and cook for 6-7 minutes.
6. Lower heat and cook for 6-8 minutes. Turn off the heat. Cool for a while.
7. Serve noodles on individual serving plates. Place tofu on top. Sprinkle lime zest and red pepper flakes and serve.

Chapter Ten: Dairy-free Ketogenic Dessert Recipes

Easy Chocolate Gelatin Pudding

Serves: 4

Ingredients:

- 2 cups canned, full fat coconut milk
- 1 teaspoon stevia powder extract
- 2 tablespoons gelatin
- 4 tablespoons cacao powder or organic cocoa
- 4 tablespoons water

Method:

1. Add cocoa, coconut milk and stevia into a pan. Place the pan over medium heat.
2. Whisk well. Add gelatin and water into a bowl and mix well.
3. Pour into the pan. Stir constantly until gelatin dissolves.
4. Turn off the heat when the mixture is warm and pour into 4 ramekins.
5. Refrigerate until it set.

Coconut Brownies

Serves:

Ingredients:

<u>For wet ingredients:</u>

- 1 cup organic birch xylitol or 4 teaspoons stevia powder extract
- 1 cup full fat coconut milk
- 2 cups coconut oil, melted
- 2 teaspoons vanilla extract
- 4 eggs

<u>For dry ingredients:</u>

- 1 ½ cups cocoa powder
- 2 cups almond flour, preferably blanched
- 1 cup shredded coconut
- 1 teaspoon baking soda
- 1 cup walnuts, chopped

Method:

1. Add all the wet ingredients into a bowl and mix well.
2. Add all the dry ingredients except walnuts into a bowl and mix well.
3. Pour the wet ingredients into the bowl of dry ingredients and mix until well combined.
4. Add walnuts and stir.

5. Pour batter into a greased, square baking dish.
6. Bake in a preheated oven at 350° F for 30-40 minutes or a toothpick, when inserted in the center, comes out clean.

Low Carb Coconut Cream with Berries

Serves: 2

Ingredients:

- 1 cup coconut cream
- 1/8 teaspoon vanilla extract
- 4 ounces fresh strawberries, chopped

Method:

1. Add all the ingredients into a bowl.
2. Blend with an immersion blender until smooth.
3. Spoon into bowls. Chill and serve.

Triple Layer Choconut Almond Butter Cups

Serves: 6

Ingredients:

For bottom layer:

- ¼ cup cacao paste, finely chopped
- ¼ teaspoon vanilla bean powder
- 2 drops pure almond extract
- 2 tablespoons coconut oil, melted
- ¼ teaspoon ground cinnamon

For middle layer:

- 2 tablespoons coconut oil, melted
- ¼ cup natural almond butter
- 1/8 teaspoon ground cinnamon

For top layer:

- ¼ cup creamy coconut butter
- 2 tablespoons coconut oil, melted

To garnish:

- A little coconut flakes, toasted
- 6 whole almonds

Method:

1. Place parchment paper cups or silicone cups in a 6-count muffin pan.
2. To make bottom layer: Add cacao paste in a microwave safe bowl and microwave on high for 20 to 30 seconds. Stir and repeat each time for 20 seconds until completely melted.
3. Add rest of the ingredients and mix well.
4. Pour into the prepared muffin pans. Place the pans in the refrigerator for 10-15 minutes or until set.
5. To make middle layer: Add all the ingredients of the middle layer into a bowl and mix well. Pour over the bottom layer in the muffin cups.
6. Place the pans in the refrigerator for 10-15 minutes or until set.
7. To make the top layer: Mix together all the ingredients of the third layer into a bowl.
8. Pour over the middle layer in the muffin cups. Place an almond in each. Sprinkle a pinch of coconut in each muffin cup.
9. Place the pans in the refrigerator for an hour.
10. Remove from the pans and place in an airtight container until use. It can last for many weeks in the refrigerator.

Raspberry Cheesecake
Serves: 8

Ingredients:

- 4.4 ounces creamed coconut milk
- ½ teaspoon vanilla extract or ¼ teaspoon vanilla bean powder
- ¼ cup almond flour
- 10 drops stevia (optional)
- ½ cup frozen raspberries
- 1 tablespoons erythritol or swerve, powdered
- 2 tablespoons coconut flour

For coating:

- 0.7 ounce cacao butter or extra virgin coconut oil
- 1.4 ounces 90% dark chocolate, unsweetened, dairy-free

Method:

1. Add creamed coconut milk, raspberries and erythritol into a blender and blend until smooth.
2. Add almond flour and coconut flour and blend until well combined.
3. Spoon into ice tray, about 1 tablespoon in each well. Freeze for an hour.
4. To make coating: Add coconut oil and dark chocolate into a heatproof bowl. Place the bowl in a double boiler. Stir occasionally until the mixture is well combined.
5. Remove the fat bombs from the ice tray and dip into the chocolate mixture.

6. Place on a tray that is lined with parchment paper. Freeze until set. Transfer into an airtight container.
7. Store in the freezer until use. It can last for many weeks in the freezer.

Pumpkin Spice Fat Bomb Ice Cream

Serves: 12

Ingredients:

- 2 cups pumpkin puree
- 8 yolks from pastured eggs
- 8 whole pastured eggs
- 2/3 cup cacao butter, melted
- ½ cup MCT oil
- 2/3 cup coconut oil
- 4 teaspoons pumpkin pie spice
- ½ cup xylitol or 30-40 drops alcohol free stevia
- Ice cubes, as required (10-15)

Method:

1. Add all the ingredients except ice cubes into a blender and blend until smooth.
2. Add 1 ice cube at a time and blend each time.
3. Pour into an ice cream maker and churn the ice cream following the manufacturer's instructions.
4. Serve immediately if you desire soft serve ice cream.
5. For firmer ice cream, transfer into a freezer safe container.
6. Freeze until firm.

7. Scoop and serve

Conclusion

Thank you once again for purchasing this book! I hope you had an enjoyable and more importantly - an informative read.

I trust this book has helped lay a strong foundation of your understanding of the dairy-free ketogenic diet. I assure you that the recipes are all tried and tested and will help you immensely in keeping your weight under control. The ingredients used in these recipes are all easily available, so you don't have to worry about cooking something with exotic ingredients. It is pretty much food cooked from your everyday ingredients.

Now that you know how to go about it, what effects you should watch out for or expect, along with the dos and don'ts of food followed by all the recipes already nudging you to step into the kitchen – you are fully prepped to venture into your dairy-free keto life.

Best wishes!

Thank you.

Bonus!

Wouldn't it be to know when Amazon's top kindle books go on Free Promotion? Well now is your chance!

I would like to give you full access to an exclusive service that will email you notifications when Amazon' top Kindle books go on Free Promotion. If you are someone who is interested in saving a ton of money, then simply go to the link below for Free access.

https://bit.ly/2xFpfOX

As a "Thank you" for downloading this book, I would like to give you "30 Day Low Carb Diet Ketosis Plan" ebook to start your keto journey.

Resources

https://draxe.com/dairy-free-diet/

https://ketodietapp.com/Blog/post/2015/01/03/Keto-Diet-Food-List-What-to-Eat-and-Avoid

https://ketoschool.com/the-43-health-benefits-of-ketogenic-dieting-in-addition-to-weight-loss-1e4ee4743f1f

https://www.medicalnewstoday.com/articles/180858.php

https://thrivestrive.com/ketosis-signs/

https://www.perfectketo.com/how-to-maintain-ketosis/

37132844R00101

Printed in Great Britain
by Amazon